Fragile Futures

Series: Epistemologies of Healing
General Editors: David Parkin and Elisabeth Hsu: both are at ISCA, Oxford

This series publishes monographs and edited volumes on indigenous (so-called traditional) medical knowledge and practice, alternative and complementary medicine, and ethnobiological studies that relate to health and illness. The emphasis of the series is on the way indigneous epistemologies inform healing, against a background of comparison with other practices, and in recognition of the fluidity between them.

Recent volumes:

Volume 22
Fragile Futures: Ambiguities of Care in Burkina Faso
Helle Samuelsen

Volume 21
Breathing Hearts: Sufism, Healing, and Anti-Muslim Racism in Germany
Nasima Selim

Volume 20
Chinese Medicine in East Africa: An Intimacy with Strangers
Elisabeth Hsu

Volume 19
Configuring Contagion: In Biosocial Epidemics
Edited by Lotte Meinert and Jens Seeberg

Volume 18
Fierce Medicines, Fragile Socialities: Grounding Global HIV Treatment in Tanzania
Dominik Mattes

Volume 17
Capturing Quicksilver: The Position, Power, and Plasticity of Chinese Medicine in Singapore
Arielle A. Smith

Volume 16
Ritual Retellings: Luangan Performances for Healing as Emergent in Practice
Isabell Herrmans

Volume 15
Healing Roots: Anthropology in Life and Medicine
Julie Laplante

Volume 14
Asymmetrical Conversations: Contestations, Circumventions, and the Blurring of Therapeutic Boundaries
Edited by Harish Naraindas, Johannes Quack and William S. Sax

Volume 13
The Body in Balance: Humoral Medicines in Practice
Edited by Peregrine Horden and Elisabeth Hsu

For a full volume listing, please see the series page on our website: https://www.berghahnbooks.com/series/epistemologies-of-healing

Fragile Futures

Ambiguities of Care in Burkina Faso

Helle Samuelsen

berghahn
NEW YORK • OXFORD
www.berghahnbooks.com

First published in 2024 by
Berghahn Books
www.berghahnbooks.com

Library of Congress Cataloging-in-Publication Data
A C.I.P. cataloging record is available from the Library of Congress
Library of Congress Cataloging in Publication Control Number: 2023053382

British Library Cataloguing in Publication Data
A catalogue record for this book is available from the British Library

ISBN 978-1-80539-197-5 hardback
ISBN 978-1-80539-259-0 epub
ISBN 978-1-80539-213-2 web pdf

https://doi.org/10.3167/9781805391975

Contents

Illustrations

Figures

Table

Acknowledgments

This book has been a long journey, and many people have contributed to its completion. First, I want to thank the citizens of Keru, Bangri, and Tenga for their hospitality, support, guidance, and engagement during my fieldwork and my many visits over more than two decades. I am thankful for the many hours they devoted to helping me understand the complexity of their everyday lives and health care practices. My warmest thanks go to Thomas, Beatrice, and their seven children, who welcomed me to their house and shared their experiences and knowledge. It has been such a rich personal experience for me and my family to follow the Bancé family, seeing the children grow up, exchanging family news, and keeping in contact, even though my visits to Burkina Faso have been restricted over the last several years because of the escalating security problems in the country. I owe my deepest gratitude to this fantastic family, including the late Jean, who guided me through the herbal landscape and introduced me to the many vernacular healers living in the area. Special thanks to the *Samadin*, members of the royal court of the Mossi king of the area, the *delegués* of the villages, and in particular the chief of Keru for giving me permission to conduct my studies in their region. I also want to thank the regional and district directors of health for taking time to talk with me and for providing me with local health data.

Furthermore, I want to thank my research assistants, Fatmata, Emmanuel, and Landry, who at different periods helped me in the field and translated between French, Bissa, and Mooré. Their dedication and commitment to the research process and fieldwork were extremely important.

I wish to thank my many research colleagues in Burkina Faso, among them Dr. Lea Paré Toé at the Institut de Recherche en Sciences de Santé (IRSS) and Professor Gabin Korbeogo, director of

Groupe de Recherche sur les Initiatives Locales (GRIL) and now director of research and head of the graduate school at the Faculty of Social Sciences at Université Joseph Ki-Zerbo in Ouagadougou. It has been a huge inspiration to jointly develop new project ideas and share project responsibilities with both. Thanks also to Professor Maxime Drabo, Research Director at IRSS and former director of Centre National de Recherche Scientifique (CNRS) in Burkina Faso, who generously shared his medical knowledge with us for the Emerging Epidemics project. I thank Dr. David Ilboudo, Dr. Yacouba Cissao, and Dr. Issa Sombié for their enthusiasm and hard work as PhD fellows in the Fragile Futures: Rural Life in Times of Conflict project. My gratitude also goes to Dr. Hamidou Sanou, Dr. Cheick Omar Diallo, and Huguette Tyenou, PhD fellow, for their flexible adjustments to fieldwork conditions during the COVID-19 pandemic and for their contributions to the Emerging Epidemics: Improving Preparedness in Burkina Faso project. I have benefited tremendously from their insights and knowledge about the functioning of the public health care system. The Danish embassy in Ouagadougou has always welcomed my visits, and the various ambassadors have shown a genuine interest in our research findings. Special thanks to Birgitte Markussen and Ulla NæsbyTawiah, both of whom served as Danish ambassadors to Burkina Faso.

I thank Professor Jean-Bernard Ouedraogo, Laboratoire d'Anthropologie des Institutions et des Organisations Sociales (LAIOS), IIAC, CNRS-EHESS for his invitation to be affiliated as a guest researcher in Paris for two periods in 2017 and 2022, as well as for his interest in discussing research findings and brainstorming new ideas. Thanks also to the Fondation Danoise, and particularly Marianne Bak Papiau, for accommodating me during research stays in Paris and to the board of Ludvig Preetzmann-Aggerholm og Hustrus Stiftelse for granting me a one-month writing retreat in Rue de la Perle.

Over the years, I have learned a lot from conversations with a number of other Scandinavian colleagues and experts on West Africa, including Sten Hagberg, Jesper Bjarnesen, Jonina Einarsdottir, Stine Loft Rasmussen, and Heidi Bojsen.

My first research project in Burkina Faso was funded by the Danish Bilharziasis Laboratory. I also received financial support from the Council for Development Research under Danida as well as the

Carlsberg Foundation, which also included two terms as by-fellow at Churchill College, University of Cambridge, UK. Two large collaborative projects—Fragile Futures: Rural Lives in Times of Conflict and Emerging Epidemics: Improving Preparedness in Burkina Faso—were both supported by grants from the Ministry of Foreign Affairs of Denmark. I want to thank the various members of the research councils and the Danish Fellowship Centre for their support and trust in our research ideas.

I am grateful to colleagues in the Health and Life Condition research group in the Department of Anthropology, University of Copenhagen, for creating a constructive and supportive academic environment. Special thanks to Professor Susan Reynolds Whyte, who knows what it means to care for students and colleagues and who continues to inspire. Thanks also to Hanne Overgaard Mogensen, Ayo Wahlberg, and Tine Gammeltoft for providing constructive feedback on my writing. To Lise Rosendal Østergaard and Pia Juul Bjertrup, my deepest thanks for their enthusiastic engagements and hard work as PhD fellows on the Fragile Futures and Emerging Epidemic projects, respectively. I have enjoyed their collaboration, friendship, and companionship in the field.

I would like to thank Britt Pinkowski Tersbøl at the Section of Global Health, University of Copenhagen, for her collegiality and friendship and for her continuous invitations to participate in projects and activities at the Global Health section. My deepest gratitude to Ib Bygbjerg, an academic and personal lighthouse, whose originality and intellectual capacity is outstanding. Thanks to Karin Schiøler and Dan Meyrowitsch for their constructive contributions as PhD supervisors in the Emerging Epidemic project.

I owe many thanks to Elisabeth Hsu and David Parkin, editors of the book series Epistemologies of Healing and to the two reviewers for their encouraging and constructive comments and suggestions, as well as to Tom Bonnington and Anthony Mason at Berghahn and to Jeremy Rehwaldt who helped with the English editing.

Last but not least, I would like to thank my family, particularly Bjarne, Anna, and Frederik, for their companionship, support, patience, and care and for continually reminding me what really matters and why.

Abbreviations

ACT: Artemisinin-based combination therapy

AIDS: Acquired Immune Deficiency Syndrome

AIS: Agent Iténerant de Santé/local health care worker

AQIM: Al Qaeda in Magreb

BAC: Baccalaureate

BCG: Bacille Calmette-Guerin vaccine

BEPC: Brevet d'études du premier cycle

CEP: Certificat d'étude primaire

CDP: Congrès pour la Démocratie et le Progrès

CDR: Comités de Défense de la Révolution/Committees for the Defense of the Revolution

CENI: Comission Électorale Nationale Indépendante

CFA: The West African CFA Franc

CNIB: Carte Nationale d'Identité Burkinabe

COVID-19: Coronavirus disease 2019

CSPS: Centre de Santé et de Promotion Sociale/dispensary

DANIDA: Denmark's development cooperation

DHS: Demographic Health Survey

DPT: Diphtheria, tetanus and pertussis vaccine

EPI: Expanded Program of Immunization

GAVI: The Vaccine Alliance

GDP: Gross Domestic Product

HIV: Human Immunodeficiency Virus

ICD: International Statistical Classification of Diseases and Related Health Problems or International Classification of Diseases

ICP: Infirmier-chef de poste/ head nurse at dispensary

INSD: Institut National de la Statistique et de la Démographie

IOM: International Organization for Migration

IPT: Intermittent preventive treatment

IRSS: Institut de Recherche en Sciences de la Santé

ISGS: Islamic State of the Greater Sahara

ITN: Insecticide-treated mosquito nets

IRS: Indoor residual spraying

MPP: Mouvement du Peuple pour le Progrès

NGO: Non-governmental organization

OCP: Onchocerciasis Control Program

OECD: Organization for Economic Co-operation and Development

OPT: Opportunistic presumptive treatment

PCR: Polymerase chain reaction

RDT: Rapid diagnostic test

REN-LAC: Le Réseau national de Lutte anti-corruption/The national anti-corruption network

UNICEF: United Nations Children's Fund

UNDP: United Nations Development Program

USAID: United States International Development

WHO: World Health Organization

Introduction

A Sudden Death

Every time I visit the village of Keru in southeastern Burkina Faso, I pass by Thomas's compound to say hello and hear the latest news from Thomas, Beatrice, and their seven children.[1] I first met them in 1996 when they all lived together in a compound just next to the marketplace. At that time, Thomas and Beatrice had five children, of whom Michel and Caroline were the youngest. Later, Beatrice gave birth to two more girls, Janine and Claudine. While I was doing fieldwork in November 2016, Caroline told me about her baby's sudden death. The sad story demonstrates how important, complex, and fragile social relationships and family bonds are in rural Burkina Faso, and it elucidates how present the spiritual world is in local care practices and in interpretations of tragedy.

After spending the morning at the district hospital interviewing the chief medical officer, my research assistant Landry and I drove to the village in the afternoon, hoping to arrange a couple of interviews for the following day. Landry was a young university student who grew up in a Bissa village not far from Keru and who spoke both Bissa and Mooré, the two main local languages spoken in this district. He was a very diligent fieldworker with a lot of empathy. We stopped as usual at Thomas and Beatrice's compound. Thomas was not at home, but his eldest son, Pascal, welcomed us into the inner courtyard to sit on the household's only two chairs. The chairs were placed in the middle of the courtyard under a small tree that provided a bit of shade against the strong sun. The customers of Beatrice's *cabaret* (millet beer bar), which she ran every third day year-round, found shade for themselves on a few wooden benches under a thatched shelter. The cabaret was located close to the entrance of the compound, near the fireplace where the *dolo* (home-brewed millet beer) was produced. On days when the cabaret was closed, we sometimes sat and talked there, but usually we were invited to the inner courtyard, which provided a little more privacy, although the two areas were divided only by a low mud wall.

As customs prescribe, we were first served a calabash of fresh water. It was a busy time of the year as the last harvest was being secured. Often, people with land work collectively in the fields all day, helping each other finish the harvest. This day, many women were working in their fields together, and other women were busy in their small vegetable gardens located outside of the village, where a nearby well provided water. Many women grew tomatoes to sell on market days when buyers from Togo or the nearby provincial town passed by. After drinking a calabash of fresh water, we were, as usual, offered a calabash of *dolo*, and Caroline sat down to talk to us. It is not unusual for married daughters to occasionally stay for a few days at their paternal compound to assist with specific tasks or participate in religious or family ceremonies. However, Thomas had told me a few days earlier that Caroline had lost her small child, who died suddenly one Sunday morning. According to Thomas, the child had not been ill prior to his death, "he just died."

Caroline was a twenty-four-year-old woman who had completed six years of education at the local school. At the age of about nineteen, she married a much older man who lived in a nearby village with his elderly mother. After the marriage, Caroline moved to live with her husband and her mother-in-law, following the patrilocal traditions in Burkina Faso. She gave birth to a girl in 2012, and three years later she gave birth to her second child, a boy, delivering him alone at home with only a little help from her mother-in-law, despite living close to a rural dispensary.

While seated in the shade under the small tree, I asked Caroline if she would tell me about the tragedy. Although ten months had passed since the death of her child, I was a bit worried and uncomfortable asking her to talk about it, but to my relief she promptly agreed. I remember Caroline, or Caro[2] as she was called by her family, from her early childhood during my initial fieldwork in Keru in 1996. At that time, she was a lively, self-confident girl with lots of energy. I often saw her playing with her younger brother Michel. As she entered adolescence, she became a shy and hard-working young woman, doing farm work and assisting with Beatrice's millet beer production. During her adult years, I had not talked much with her; she always kept to herself, staying inside, I surmised, because she had suffered a serious corneal infection and strong sunlight caused her pain. However, on this occasion, it was as if she really wanted to tell her story. I sensed a great sadness but also a kind of vacillation. It was clear that she felt locked into a situation: she could not continue living with her husband, yet moving back with her parents did not seem to be a viable solution either. She wanted me to understand her situation, and perhaps she hoped that I would be able to help her. She sat on a small stool just in front of us. To my surprise she started to disclose her story in French—I had never before heard her speak much in French. But this time, she spoke French during most of the heartbreaking interview, only switching to Mooré in the last part of the conversation. Her statements, which revealed how complex family relations can be, were very clear:

> *Helle*: Last year you gave birth at home and the baby was fine. How did your boy die?
>
> *Caro*: He just died like that. He was not ill before he died. He just died.
>
> *Helle*: He just died? He had not been ill before he died?
>
> *Caro*: No, he was not ill before he died. It was a Sunday, he died. I woke up Sunday morning and went to church with him.
>
> *Helle*: Did you go to church in this village or in the village where you live?
>
> *Caro*: Yes, at that village, at Bangri. At the prayers there, I breastfed him. He was not dead then. It was after the prayers. I placed the child on my back, and we went home. It was when coming home that I saw that the child had died. He had simply died, just like that.

According to Caro, the cause of the child's death was related to a conflict with her husband and mother-in-law, an active woman, probably in her mid-eighties, whom I had met a couple of times. Caro explained:

> *Caro*: The problem is that my husband is Muslim, and I am Christian. He has told me that if I take the child to the church, the child will die. His mother, my mother-in-law, has also forbidden me to go to church with the child, saying that in that case, he will die. My husband says that it is his child, and that the child is therefore Muslim, and that it is not my child. I have replied that it is also my child. I have said to my husband that the child belongs to both of us. The mother of my husband has talked with "things." I don't know how to explain this. My mother-in-law has

> performed some sacrifices to the ancestors in order for the child to die. She has told me that if I go to church with the child, he will die. She has sacrificed the child to the ancestors of her natal village. My mother-in-law has told me that she does not agree with me to convert the child to Christianity, as she is herself Muslim. But my mother-in-law is herself Christian, as she has done the catechist, and she is baptized. That day, both of us went to church. When my mother-in-law went [to her village] to do the sacrifice, she told me that my child would die on my back.

Caro was clearly worried about the conflict with her husband and her in-laws, and she was afraid that the mother-in-law would also bewitch her four-year-old daughter. I will unfold the story of the sudden death of Caro's son in more detail in chapter 2, as it illustrates the importance of the spiritual world in interpretations of a child's sudden death in this part of Burkina Faso and highlights that caring for a small child and caring for family relations are sometimes at odds.

Aim of the Book

The aim of this book is to illustrate how rural citizens of Burkina Faso encounter and live with a fragile state and an elusive public health care system. At a time when medical anthropologists focus, to a large extent, on biomedicine, with clinics or hospitals serving as the main field sites (Hannig 2017; Livingston 2012; McKay 2017; Scherz 2018; Street 2014; Strong 2020; Wendland 2010), this book follows Dorothy Hodgson's recommendation to engage in research with long-marginalized rural peoples. Hodgson argues that "perspectives and experiences 'from the margins' offer key theoretical and political insights into this complicated place we call 'Africa' by challenging grand narratives of modernization, of 'Africa rising,' of supposedly 'universal' ideas of progress and justice" (Hodgson 2017: 38). The chronically precarious political and social situations of countries like Burkina Faso raise a number of questions: How do rural citizens perceive and relate to an "absent-present" state? How do they balance the insecurities and uncertainties of everyday life with the search for new opportunities to improve their lives as well as the lives of their relatives? How do rural citizens exercise hope and agency in the quest for health care? How do they relate to and imagine the state? *Fragile Futures* is based on more than twenty years of engagement with Burkina Faso and, in particular, on my engagement with the Bancé family. Their story discloses the hardships, ambiguities, hopes, and ambitions of populations in low-income rural societies. Each of the chapters includes narratives from members of the family.

Ambiguities of Care

Throughout this book, I use the term *ambiguities of care* to frame understandings of care, illness, and treatment seeking. Ambiguity refers to "the quality of being open to more than one interpretation" (Oxford English Dictionary 2008), and it is this "openness" that I find particularly interesting. Sickness itself is an ambiguous state, and one central task of caring is the management of this ambiguity (Holden and Littlewood 2015: 170). Families experience ambiguities of care when a child falls sick and decisions have to be made about how best to intervene. Each new step of the therapeutic pathway is impelled by uncertainty, but also incites hope for healing and restoration of everyday life. The decision about whom to consult in case of sickness is ambiguous. It is, I argue, not so much a choice between different epistemologies, but a pragmatic choice of time and cost and a choice about how best to confirm and nurture good relations with human as well as non-human beings. The symptomatology of a disease such as malaria is itself ambiguous, and getting a negative result from a rapid diagnostic test for malaria at the rural dispensary and then receiving a prescription for malaria medicine from the same nurse is also an ambiguous experience. As I elaborate later, this seemingly illogical praxis relates to the fact that Burkina Faso has a strong focus on the fight against malaria, and the diagnostic repertoire of the nurses at the dispensaries is limited.

Taking *ambiguities of care* as an analytical framework for exploring different forms of care relationships, I wish to illustrate, in line with China Scherz's study from Kampala (Scherz 2018), that if we want to understand the diversity of human practice and experience within the domain of health, we need a renewed focus on treatment seeking in medical anthropology that includes both vernacular healing by local experts and self-treatment at home. In this book, I argue that families, and in particular mothers of small children, spend an enormous amount of time on care work. Taking care of family members is both about managing actual cases of sickness in the most appropriate (and economically sound) ways and about maintaining and nurturing various social relationships to humans and nonhuman beings. My core contention is that citizens of Keru actively and intelligently address the ambiguities of sickness and care and explore potentials and openings in their determination to maintain and secure a decent future for themselves and their families.

Fragility refers to being easily broken or damaged, being delicate and vulnerable. At the social level, fragility is related to other concepts such as uncertainty, insecurity, contingency, and vulnerability. While these concepts are interrelated, it might be useful to distinguish between them in order to see how they relate to and complement each other. In her epilogue to *Dealing with Uncertainty in Contemporary African Lives*, edited by Liv Haram and Bawa Yamba (Haram and Yamba 2009), Susan Reynolds Whyte defines uncertainty, insecurity, and contingency, and she briefly discusses how these concepts feed into and are often entangled with each other (Whyte 2009: 213–15). Uncertainty, she says, may be thought of as a state of mind and minding. It pertains to our situated concerns and "refers to a lack of absolute knowledge: inability to predict the outcome of events or to establish facts about phenomena and connections with assurance" (Whyte 2009: 213). Uncertainty is a way of thinking about the future, and it creates worries and fears. In Whyte's definition, insecurity denotes a social condition where there is "a lack of protection from dangers, weakness in the social arrangements that provide some kind of safety net when adversity strikes" (Whyte 2009: 214). Having little room to maneuver may generate uncertainty. Contingency is related to the two abovementioned concepts but refers more specifically to an existential situation. To be contingent "is to be dependent on, or affected by, *something else* that cannot be fully foreseen or controlled" (Whyte 2009: 214). Contingency is about the unexpected, the events that may arise suddenly and affect one's plans for the future. All three concepts relate to the present and the future: uncertainty refers to a state of mind, insecurity to a social situation, and contingency to an existential situation. However, they all take their point of departure from an existing situation entailing negative consequences for the future.

According to Whyte, dealing with uncertainty is not so much about trying to make things certain as about trying to create more security. While insecurity and contingency are very closely related, contingency emphasizes dependency and interrelatedness. Vulnerability, which is also about dependency, is closely related to contingency but denotes a social situation. The concept of vulnerability is used by social welfare institutions and aid agencies to categorize people—such as orphans or malnourished children—with extra needs or entitlements due to their exposure to particular risks (Whyte 2009: 215). My use of *fragility* as a concept relates closely to the notion of contingency, as it also accentuates interdependence. Within the anthropology of philosophy, Paul Ricoeur relates fragility very closely to interdependency and responsibility. Ricoeur sees the human being not as an autonomous, independent individual but as an individual dependent on other people, constantly balancing definite and infinite desires while striving for the good life (Ricoeur 1986; Schaafsma 2014: 163). While Ricoeur has been an important figure within philosophy and the human sciences, there is now a growing interest in his work within the social sciences, particularly among scholars working with "narratives" and "pragmatism" (Borisenkova 2012; Schaafsma 2014; Van Nistelrooij, Schaafsma, and Tronto 2014). Ricoeur's strong focus on the fundamental importance of social relationships for the individual human being is in line with the perspective of social anthropology (Carney 2015; Kearney 1996; Ricoeur 1994). In "Fragility and Responsibility," Ricoeur elaborates on the importance (and the imperative) of "responsibility," giving the example of the birth of a child. He writes:

> Consider the birth of a child—its mere existence obliges. We are rendered responsible by the fragile. Yet, what does "rendered responsible" mean? When the fragile is not something but someone—an individual, groups, communities, even humanity—this someone appears to us, entrusted to our care, placed in our custody. Let us be careful, however. The image of custody or the burden, which one takes upon oneself, should not render us inattentive to the other component emphasized by the expression "entrusted to our care"—the fragile as "someone" who relies on us, expects our assistance and care and trusts that we shall fulfill our obligations. This bond of trust is fundamental. (Ricoeur 1996: 16)

Ricoeur's analysis of the intrinsic relations between fragility, care, and responsibility informs my work. In Keru, everyday health care activities, both preventive and therapeutic, take place in a fragile environment where each individual is, ontologically speaking, fragile.

People are connected through interdependent social relationships with other human beings as well as non-human beings, and this interdependency is expressed in the everyday, pragmatic practices of caregiving, where family members invest in the future of their children, family, kin, and community. Ricoeur's notion of fragility resonates particularly well with my ethnographic analysis because it "directs us towards the future of a being in need of help to survive and to grow" (Ricoeur and Kearney 1996: 16). Interdependency and responsibility are also about caring, understood in both a practical and an affective sense. The notion of care also has a temporal dimension: to care for someone is to engage in actions directed toward the future. Caring for a child seeks to ensure the child's growth, and caring for a sick person fosters a process of healing.

Potentialities and Hope

In this ethnography, *ambiguity* refers to the multiple uncertainties, contingencies, and potentialities that disrupt everyday life but that also continuously provide openings and offer hope (Hage 2003; Millar 2014; Vigh 2008, 2011; Zigon 2018). Conditions of fragility and uncertainty are not only negative; they include the potential for new opportunities, the hope of a different future. The notion of hope has a number of connotations, such as desiring, wishing, wanting, waiting, and dreaming. To understand the texture of everyday life in Keru, I explore the relations between fragility, care work, and hope. As I show in the following chapters, the citizens of Keru continuously assess possibilities, seize opportunities, and take chances in their determination to negotiate and form their own futures and those of their families. Fragility, care, and hope include both social and temporal dimensions; they all "express in one way or another modes in which human beings relate to their future" (Hage 2003: 10). Societal hope, as Ghassan Hage (with inspiration from Pierre Bourdieu) defines it, is allocated through social opportunities or social routes by which individuals can define a meaningful and dignified social life: "If hope is the way we construct a meaningful future for ourselves . . . such futures are only possible within society, because society is the distributor of social opportunities for self-realization. We can call this hope societal hope" (2003: 15). The distribution of hope is, for Hage, an intrinsic quality of any society, maintaining the possibility of upward social mobility—nursing dreams of better education, jobs, and lifestyles, even when those dreams often remain unrealized.

Precarious and uncertain living conditions can also be used to negotiate and explore opportunities and alternative futures. Hope is a means to imagine a future that is then projected back into the present to influence the best possible route toward that future (S. Turner 2015; Vigh 2009). Hopefulness is "a disposition to be confident in the face of the future, to be open to it and welcoming to what it will bring, even if one does not know for sure what it will bring" (Hage quoted in S. Turner 2015: 175). This complex task of balancing the present with hope for the future is a fundamental component of agency and of being en route. As Ricoeur formulates it: "I must hope in order to believe that I am able to act" (Dauenhauer 1986: xv). In the chapters that follow, I examine different modes of fragility and uncertainty with specific focus on the various practices and actions that express hope and hopefulness.

Faced with a weak and elusive health infrastructure, many citizens, both rural and urban, feel neglected by the state and mistrust of the government has been growing; yet, the state–citizen relationship is ambiguous, because "the state continues to exercise a 'crucial presence' as an 'object of desire'" (Street 2012: 16). Thus, I explore ambiguities of care in different types of relationships. I focus on the caregiver–patient relationships at the household level, where family members continually have to make decisions about how best to prevent and treat sickness. In therapeutic engagements, families choose between and consult different types of healing experts, each of whom proposes meaningful therapeutic pathways, but with no pregiven guarantee of positive outcomes. When patients and their families consult the dispensary or the district hospital, the care practices provide patients with some kind of security, but the routinization and the limited diagnostic repertoire also disclose how fragile the system is. I show how rural citizens, through their engaged and active care practices, continuously work with the ambiguities that sickness brings, and I argue that conditions of fragility and uncertainty can be productive, because they open up new opportunities. However, hope is, as Jarrett Zigon argues, not only and always about striving toward a new and better future, but it is also about the perseverance of a sane and decent life. Hope is thus also about maintaining the world as it has been lived through, and hope is what enjoins us to 'keep going'" (Zigon 2018: 71–72). Pragmatic "trying again" and persistent tinkering are gestures of care that actively attend to openings and potentialities in the search for a sane life (Zigon 2018). Following specific cases of sickness and listening to (particularly) mothers' reflections about their therapeutic options and decisions, I trace how hopes, worries, and disappointments unfold over time.

Structural Fragility

The term *fragility* has also been used widely within development discourse to categorize states. The characterization of Burkina Faso as a "fragile state" or, perhaps more precisely, a state with "limited statehood" (Börzel and Risse 2021) is relevant for the discussion of fragility and hope in a rural community as well as for understanding rural citizens' relations to the state.

Originally, the donor community identified a rather broad and heterogeneous group of countries as fragile. As Jörg Faust, Jörn Grävingholt, and Sebastian Ziaja (2015) explain, "fragility" summarizes various features of weak, decaying, failed, failing, or otherwise defunct states. Fragility as a concept, with roots in political theories of state formation, was taken up by policymakers when they were confronted with government failures in Haiti and Somalia. Although the original definition of a "fragile state" is not absolutely clear, there seems to be common agreement that fragile states, or states with "limited statehood," are unable to control violence, address popular demands for representation, or guarantee minimal living standards (Faust et al. 2015: 411). Burkina Faso was ranked 37 of 178 countries on the 2020 Fragility State Index and mentioned as one of the five countries whose condition had worsened the most over the previous year.[3] Yemen was first on the list, identified as the most fragile state in the world. The ranking is based on twelve vulnerability indicators grouped in four categories: cohesion, social, economic, and political. Burkina has the worst score on "security apparatus" (8.7 where 10 is the maximum), "demographic pressure" (8.6), and "public service" (8.4). The public service indicator, the one most directly relevant to providing health care, is defined in the following way:

> The Public Services Indicator refers to the presence of basic state functions that serve the people. On the one hand, this may include the provi-

> sion of essential services, such as health, education, water and sanitation, transport infrastructure, electricity and power, and internet and connectivity. On the other hand, it may include the state's ability to protect its citizens, such as from terrorism and violence, through perceived effective policing. Further, even where basic state functions and services are provided, the Indicator further considers to whom—whether the state narrowly serves the ruling elites, such as security agencies, presidential staff, the central bank, or the diplomatic service—while failing to provide comparable levels of service to the general populace—such as rural versus urban populations. The Indicator also considers the level and maintenance of general infrastructure to the extent that its absence would negatively affect the country's actual or potential development.[4]

The fact that the public service score is so high indicates that the capacity to deliver the most basic services, including health care, is very low. The Fragile States Index has issued a "warning" for Burkina Faso, just one level below the "alert" issued for the most fragile states.[5]

Burkina Faso's economy grew at an average of more than 5 percent annually between 1991 and 2016. However, the notion of "Africa rising," used to characterize the rather impressive economic growth of many African countries, does not apply to the living conditions in rural Burkina Faso. The country's economy relies heavily on agriculture—around 70 to 80 percent of the population is employed in this sector, mostly as subsistence farmers. Burkina Faso is a landlocked country with few natural resources. Cotton is the main cash crop, and gold exports play an increasingly important role in the country's economy. Unfortunately, the government has not managed to improve the living conditions of its people significantly, and many still live in absolute poverty. Burkina Faso is consistently ranked near the bottom of the UNDP Human Development Index.[6] In 2016, the country was ranked 185 of 188 countries, with 46 percent of the population below the poverty line (Zeilig 2017).[7] In 1996, when I started fieldwork in Burkina Faso, the total population was estimated at around 10.5 million; in 2020, it was estimated to be more than 19 million. Such a population increase puts a lot of pressure on land resources, the political system, and individual families.[8]

In 2014, Blaise Compaoré, who had been president since 1987, wanted to change the constitution so he could continue for yet another term as president. However, the proposed change stirred up protests and resistance against Compaoré and his brother, who also had a prominent position in the government. A widespread *insurrection Populaire* (popular uprising) was organized by the *Balai citoyen* (broom citizen) movement led by a famous Burkinabe musician in collaboration with trade unions and other civil society organizations (Hagberg et al. 2015). Demonstrations, strikes, and other protests took place during the uprising in the major cities, but some demonstrations also took place in regional towns. Blaise Compaoré was exiled to Côte d'Ivoire, and he apparently managed to escape with cars loaded with "state money." After a short-lived military coup in September 2015, fresh elections were held in November 2015. Roch Marc Kaboré, a prominent figure in Compaoré's government until ten months prior to the elections, won the first round with more than 53 percent of the vote. Hopes were high that democracy in Burkina Faso would be revitalized and that the precarious living conditions of the majority of the population would finally be addressed.

Although many citizens, including many in Keru, expressed their disappointment with Roch Kaboré's government, he was reelected in November 2020. However, his time as president was short. In January 2022, Colonel Paul-Henri Damiba staged a military coup and installed himself as the leader of an interim government. He accused the sitting government of not being able to provide security in the country. Only eight months later, another coup d'état took place and

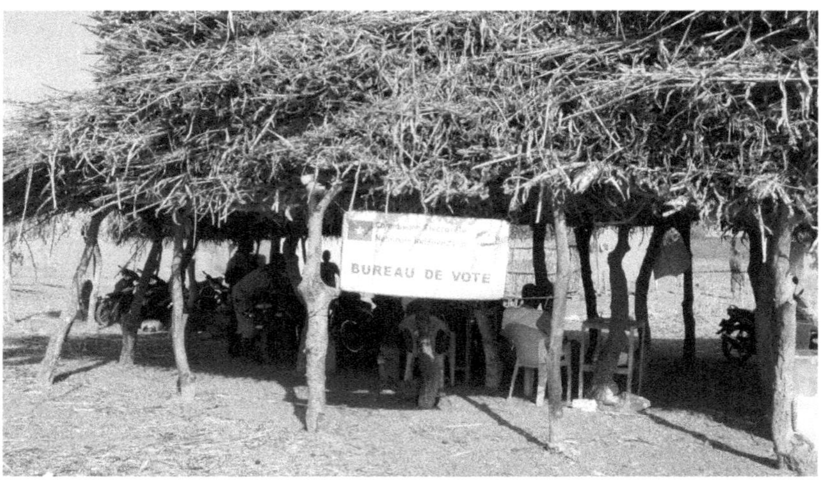

Figure 0.1. Polling Station in a rural area, Burkina Faso (© Helle Samuelsen 2023)

Damiba was removed. This time, Captain Ibrahim Traoré, who originally supported Damiba's coup, took power. He accused Damiba of being more concerned with politics than with fighting the jihadists in order to restore peace in the country.

Instability and insecurity characterize several countries in West Africa. Political conflicts in Côte d'Ivoire, particularly during the period from 2012 to 2014 and during more recent presidential elections, have brought to the surface fundamental ethnic and regional tensions. The borders to Burkina Faso were temporarily closed during a political crisis in 2014, the economy of Côte d'Ivoire slowed down, and many Burkinabe migrants returned home during the crisis with little chance of finding a job at home. The security situation in the Central Sahel, including Mali, Burkina Faso, and Niger, has been particularly tense since 2014. The political conflict in Mali, where jihadists have controlled the northern part of the country for several years, revealed the weakness in the country's democratic government, and the military coup in 2020 exposed the volatility of the current situation. In Burkina Faso, terrorist attacks, mainly by AQIM (Al Qaeda in Magreb), Ansaroul Islam, and the Islamic State of the Greater Sahara (ISGS), have become more frequent. The jihadist groups no longer restrict their activities to the border areas in the northern part of the Sahel, where the security situation has long been delicate, as had been their strategy for years (Hagberg et al. 2019). In January 2016, bomb blasts took place at a hotel and a café in Burkina Faso's capital, Ouagadougou. Both places were known as hubs for Western tourists and aid workers. Serious attacks on military barracks, public schools, health facilities, and civilians have increased since 2016. Kidnappings of national citizens and foreigners have occurred in Mali and Burkina Faso in recent years. The Ebola epidemic in Guinea, Sierra Leone, and Liberia shattered the countries' economies and revealed how weak and vulnerable their health care systems were. All three are among the poorest countries in the world. West Africa, in other words, is politically tense and economically fragile, and understanding this is important for my analysis of everyday life and health care in rural Burkina Faso.

The combination of a rapidly growing population and the majority of the population surviving on subsistence agriculture places rural families in Burkina Faso under pressure. With few natural resources, political unrest in the region, high unemployment rates in urban areas, and a weak government barely able to deliver even the most basic services, most people are left to fend for themselves. Many families depend on remittances from their relatives among the nearly 1.6 million migrant workers who move to other countries in the region or abroad to work in the agricultural or service sectors. The most important destinations are Côte d'Ivoire, Ghana, Mali, Niger, Italy, Benin, France, Nigeria, Gabon, and Germany.[9] In Keru, most families include one or more migrant workers, and many women and children depend on the often unstable remittances they send home. However, far from all migrants experience success. During my visit to the village in 2014, in the midst of conversations about the proposed changes to the constitution, the Bancé family was discussing whether to send Michel, at the time nineteen years old, abroad, as local options for finding work or making a living in subsistence agriculture were very limited.

This book, *Fragile Futures*, is about both fragile relationships and fragile institutions. It is about the fragility of lives in rural Burkina Faso, where people depend on and are responsible to each other, care for each other, and worry about their own futures as well as the futures of their children. It is also about people's experience of hope as they look for opportunities, seize possibilities, and anticipate that the state will take up the responsibility of providing basic services, including improved health care, to all Burkinabes. *Fragile Futures* is about the ambiguities of sickness, care, and seeking treatment in rural Burkina Faso. It is about the everyday life and about the ordinary and relentless care required to keep children healthy. It is about mothers' paths in and out of biomedical state institutions and their use of local, informal health care providers.

The Absent-Present State

Looking at the Burkina state over recent decades, we see at least three paradoxes. First, Blaise Compaoré's presidency, which lasted twenty-seven years, was both weak and strong. Second, the government, at both the local and national levels, is stable and fragile at the same time. Third, the state is simultaneously absent from and present in people's lives (Law 2002; Masquelier 2001; Street 2012).

The first paradox relates to the fact that Compaoré's presidency had been quite strong until 2014. He was elected and reelected several times, and, during his rule, he managed to steer clear of a number of conflicts between ethnic groups inside the country, balancing the power of the government with that of the traditional chiefs. Furthermore, he succeeded in negotiating "peace deals" with jihadist groups in the north and west by offering them certain privileges. In addition, the economy grew, but that growth did not benefit the rural poor, who were largely ignored by the government.

The country's health policy, which, since the signing of the Alma-Ata Declaration in 1978, has been characterized by a long-standing focus on district-based primary health care, highlights a second paradox, this one about the stability and fragility of governance. Despite a number of successes, such as high vaccination rates, a reduction in the average distance to public health facilities, and the introduction of the rapid diagnostic test for malaria, the health care system continues to face huge challenges in delivering basic services and quality care (Melberg et al. 2016). The third paradox—that the state is both absent and present—is conspicuous in the rural parts of the country. The notion of the absent-present state is central to my analysis of health care practices and the use of the public health facilities in rural Burkina Faso. I draw here on John Law's definition of the "absent-present." In his analysis of aircraft stories, he describes heterogeneity: "How it is that whatever is not there is also there. How that which is there is also not there. Both/and rather than either/or. Or both/and either/or and both/and. Heterogeneity, then, is about the differences that reside in connection and disconnection. Or, more precisely, it is about the ambivalent distributions entailed in dis/connection" (Law 2002: 96). As in the case of the aircraft brochures Law analyzed, where the technical descriptions of the aircraft included both an absence and a presence of "the real world," of "what actually happens" (Law 2002: 95–99), so too do state-governed rural health facilities include both absences and presences. Government buildings, such as schools, dispensaries, and prefectures, dot the landscape with their distinctive architecture, but they are remarkably empty of both people and equipment. The physical facility is there, but it is at the same time characterized by material absence, as in the case of health facilities, basic diagnostic equipment is usually unavailable or broken, and basic elements of infrastructure, such as running water, stable electricity, and toilet facilities, are absent.

As I show in my analysis of the medical field and the services provided by the local dispensary (chapter 6), another type of absence-presence also emerges in the health care system. While the health care policy of Burkina Faso clearly states that rural dispensaries serve as the first point of contact with the government health care system, patients are often uncertain about how much to pay for the services, whether health workers will listen and understand, and whether the diagnoses and therapies provided will secure recovery from illness (thus proving that the visit was "worth the money"). Patients bring these unspoken questions with them, but they do not fit into the algebra of health policy.[10]

In this book, I look at the presence—and absence—of "the state" in everyday life, focusing particularly on how the rural citizens of Keru and neighboring villages managed their lives in the context of an "absent-present" state. Within the social sciences scholars have produced a substantial literature (and corresponding debate) on the definition of the state and the role of the state in the context of a globalized world (Adebanwi 2022; Blom Hansen and Stepputat 2001; Bouchard 2011; Das and Poole 2004; Engberg-Pedersen, Andersen, and Stepputat 2008; Ferguson 2006; Inda and Rosaldo 2002; OECD 2010; Sharma and Gupta 2006; Street 2012). I primarily subscribe to an analysis of the state as a cultural constitution—that is, as Aradhana Sharma and Akhil Gupta (2006: 11) formulate it: "how people perceive the state, how their understandings are shaped by their particular locations and intimate and embodied encounters with state process and officials and how the state manifests itself in their lives." This approach implies an investigation of everyday practices during which citizens encounter representatives of the state, whether they are standing in line for vaccinations at the health center, participating in a public meeting at the local school, or filing a complaint about a neighbor at the office of the *préfet*. The state is substantiated through these banal bureaucratic practices, usually located in a set of institutions (Sharma and Gupta 2006).

In one sense, this is a book about people living at the margins of the state—or rather about how marginal the state seems to be to many rural citizens. It is a state that, on the one hand, sees its role as creating order and, in a Foucauldian sense, works hard to control the population (Foucault 2007, 2012; Scott 1998). On the other hand, it is a state that has neither the means nor the will to secure a "bare"

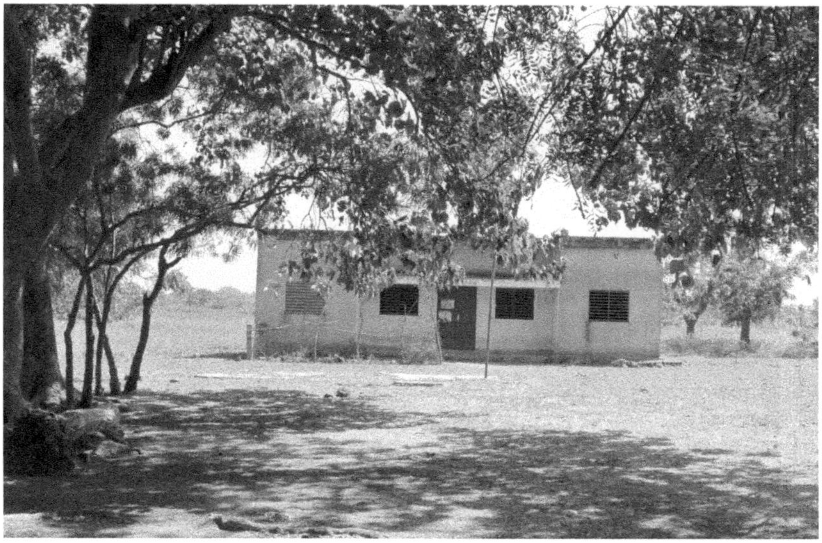

Figure 0.2. Municipal office in a rural area, Burkina Faso (© Helle Samuelsen 2023)

life for its citizens (Agamben 1998). The "absent-present" state is marginal to the everyday life of those in rural villages. The citizens of Keru experience the representatives of the state as strangers. This becomes particularly clear when they enter the dispensary or hospital. Here they are almost silent, speaking only when addressed directly, and their approach to the public health staff is usually very humble.

In a simple spatial sense, the villages are geographically marginal, located far from the capital, where the main government and business centers are located. The network of roads, electrical service, public water supplies, and other infrastructure becomes thinner and thinner the greater the distance from the capital of Ouagadougou; often the quality of those services becomes poorer and poorer as well. Alice Street's description of "weak" or "absent-present" states in her work on Madang Hospital in Papua New Guinea resonates very well with the situation in Burkina Faso. In Papua New Guinea, Street notes, "the state exists primarily as an absence. The state is not imagined as an abstract entity but as an urban elite of politicians and administrators who have little interest in bringing governance, and associated 'development,' to the nation's rural inhabitants" (Street 2012: 16).

In Keru, state institutions related to education, health care, and local government are visible, but few services are available. Mothers with small children queue up early in the morning on vaccination days at the dispensary in Tenga, which serves about twelve villages, but nurses confirmed that few patients turn up for other consultations. Not only was the dispensary almost empty of people, it was also empty of instruments and essential utilities such as running water and latrines. The classrooms at the local school provide wooden benches for the pupils and a table for the teacher, as well as a large blackboard. However, there are no books or other supplies; the children have to bring their own notebooks and "Bics" (pens). The lack of services has continued from my first trip to Keru in 1996 until the present, despite the village's growth.

State institutions, even those located in the village, feel distant from the experience of everyday people. Staff are frequently absent from their posts. Often, the prefect and mayor attend meetings in the district headquarters, and many of the government staff drive to the nearest town in the afternoon, where their families and friends may live, as few of them are locals themselves. The architecture of the government buildings clearly signifies that they represent the state. The square buildings with cement floors and tin roofs, built with proper bricks, stand out from the village's round mud-brick houses with thatched roofs, though local architecture increasingly resembles that of the government buildings. At the school, most of the teaching is conducted in French, the official language of Burkina Faso, although most children speak Mooré or Bissa at home. In the last chapter, I shift focus from rural Burkina Faso to an analysis of urban responses to the COVID-19 pandemic in Burkina Faso with a particular focus on how the state–citizen relationship was temporarily affected by the lockdown and the understandings of COVID-19 as an exceptional disease.

Biopower

In Keru, most people believed that the recent economic progress of the country had benefited only the urban elites. Both men and women in the village explained how difficult it was to make enough income from subsistence farming or small-scale trading to sustain and care for their families. Hage explains the role of nation-states:

"Nation-states are supposed to be capable of providing a nurturing and caring environment," and if citizens are "cared for," citizens "care back" through their active and affective participation in the nation (Hage 2003: 29–30). That was not happening in Keru. Understanding the fragility of Burkina Faso's government—partly due to a weak economy and an unstable government and partly due to massive security threats from jihadist groups operating in Central Sahel—is important for getting a sense of how citizens in Keru as well as in a city like Bobo-Dioulasso imagine and relate to the state and its services.

In addition to their experience of economic marginality, many people in Keru were disappointed in politicians. They expressed concern about the dominance of the Mossi people in government and other powerful positions. The village (and other parts of the Boulgou province) is primarily inhabited by Bissa, and the tense relationship between the Bissa and the Mossi, the major ethnic group in the country, has a long history. The Bissa claim that they were the first to settle in this area, later providing some land to the Mossi. However, the Mossi have always been politically strong with powerful kingdoms throughout Burkina Faso. A Mossi king continues to rule through the traditional chieftain system in Tenkodogo, and he is supported by both Mossi and Bissa people of the region through various gifts in return for different forms of protection. However, in recent years, the tensions between the groups have escalated, particularly concerning land and water use (Cissao 2019; Korbeogo 2013), and some villages now have both a Bissa and a Mossi chief.

Inspired by Veena Das and her colleagues (Das and Poole 2004), I explore the relationship between the margin, in this case the experience of everyday life in Keru, and the representations of the state.[11] I am particularly interested in how "technologies of power" are practiced and perceived within the domain of health service provision. This is not a simple relationship since many of the conventional technologies of power do not work well in Burkina Faso. The state attempts to "manage" the rural population in various ways, while at the same time failing or neglecting to provide the most basic public goods. In the chapter on COVID-19, I examine the ambiguous local responses to the many restrictions introduced by the government and show how the imposition of the lockdown as a technology of power was praised by some urban residents—at least temporarily.

Veena Das and Deborah Poole discuss marginality and relations to the state noting, that "the state is continually both experienced and undone through the *illegibility* of its own practices" (Das and Poole 2004: 10) when the state resorts to illegible acts, such as corruption or falsification of documents. Although the health sector in Burkina Faso is characterized by extensive corruption, or irregular administration (REN-LAC 2018), I will not here focus directly on how the state and its representatives establish laws and engage in illegible practices. However, the underlying discussion of authority is relevant for this book. Max Weber describes three basic types of authority: legal, traditional, and charismatic (Weber 1978: 215). Bureaucratic organizations, such as public health facilities, are ideally built on legal authority. They are rational, set up to perform specific tasks. Weber explains how offices, statuses, and roles within a bureaucracy are clearly defined and hierarchically organized with specific and precise rules and regulations guiding the work of bureaucrats. As a result of the rules governing practice, bureaucrats are expected to be impersonal in their work, treating others fairly and objectively in all situations (Weber 1978). Bureaucratic organizations are thus contrasted with systems based on traditional or charismatic authority. When focusing on the margins, the notion of authority becomes central. How do members of the "local bureaucracy" perform their authority? How do the rural citizens relate to this type of authority—and to other forms of authority, such as the traditional authority enacted by the local chiefdoms (Pare Toe and Samuelsen 2020)?

Das and Poole also study the margin as the space between bodies, law, and discipline in which biopower is produced (Das and Poole 2004: 9–10). *Biopower* and *biopolitics* have become key terms in contemporary theorizing about the interface between biomedicine, the biological body, and politics. This discussion takes its point of departure in Michel Foucault's work on the role of statistics, population counts, and other regulations in the modern state, where the emphasis has shifted from the sovereignty of the state over territories to the state's management of human life (Das and Poole 2004; Foucault 2012; Samuelsen and Steffen 2004). As I discuss in chapter 6, metrics, based on standard reporting formats, play an important role in the government's health care policy and its continuous focus on the fight against malaria.

The capacity to perform medical sovereignty on biological bodies is limited. Government health care professionals have neither the skills nor the technologies to accommodate the biomedical and bureaucratic agenda of government institutions. The institutions are the loci for biopower, but they are relatively weak. The relationship between the state and the margin moves in two directions. The health staff (or other government employees), who have the authority to be in command and manage the medical treatment of patients, depend not only on having the relevant technologies to execute their power but also on being recognized and visible to patients as professional experts with decisive capacities for action. In turn, patients struggle to make their bodies seen by the health care professionals. This interdependent relationship of "rights and duties" is analyzed by Adriana Petryna in her study of life after Chernobyl, where people affected by the catastrophe accept their duties as citizens but also claim their rights as biological citizens and seek disability entitlements (Petryna 2013a). In chapter 7, I return to the discussion of biopower and the rights and duties of the state to take care of its citizens.

The question of "rights and duties" is also taken up by Vinh-Kim Nguyen in his discussion of therapeutic citizenship in relation to the AIDS epidemic in West Africa, where it became important to recruit HIV-positive patients for various treatment trials. Being part of a treatment trial implies certain rights, such as the right to medicine and the right to food aid (Nguyen 2010; Samuelsen 2016). Likewise, Susan Reynolds Whyte, Michael Whyte, Lotte Meinert, and Jennipher Twebaze explore therapeutic clientship in the relationship between clients and an AIDS care program in Uganda, where the participants, by joining the program, gained access to new benefits and opportunities (Whyte et al. 2013). Nguyen's and Whyte's research does not directly examine the relationship between citizens and the state; rather, they consider the relationships between citizens and nongovernmental organizations, because such groups often fill the gap left by states unable or unwilling to act.

In *Fragile Futures*, I unfold the complex relationships between health authorities and citizens in Keru with a specific focus on how rural citizens manage illness and treatment under circumstances where little professional biomedical health care is available. In the last chapter, I examine the exception: how the government managed to deploy biopower during the COVID-19 pandemic—and how urban citizens responded to these powerful interventions. *Fragile Futures* is in conversation with anthropological literature on global health, where "local" ethnographic studies are combined with critical questions about the role of security, politics, and power (Adams 2016; Adebanwi 2022; Biehl and Petryna 2013; Bierschenk and de Sardan 2014; Das and Han 2015; de Sardan 2008, 2015; Farmer 1999, 2006; Holmes 2013; Manderson, Smith-Morris et al. 2010; Nguyen 2010; Team and Manderson 2020; Van der Geest and Whyte 1988; Wilkinson and Kleinman 2016). I explore how "ordinary" care practices in rural Burkina Faso are shaped by household, community, and national politics within the political and economic framework of an unstable state. With the notion of the "absent-present state" (Law 2002; Street 2012, 2014). I show that the state is indeed present in people's perceptions despite its elusiveness or absence in their everyday life.

Anthropological Engagement

Fragile Futures builds on more than twenty years of engagement with Burkina Faso and particularly on fieldwork in three villages in a southeastern province. Throughout my work in Burkina, I have remained in contact with the Bancé family in the village of Keru. This close contact has allowed me to follow the ups and downs of this family and the village where they live. During fieldwork periods, I have followed the everyday life in the village; at other times, I have been absent for long periods and even more eager to catch up at the next visit. In other words, I do not claim to have in-depth knowledge about village life during the whole period, but returning to the village again and again has given me a sense of continuity.

This book is a response to the call for "slow research" by Vincanne Adams, Nancy J Burke, and Ian Whitmarsh (2014). The slow research movement argues for a change of research perspectives, particularly in relation to global health, that pays increased attention to local specificities: "Slow research takes the local as a starting point. It calls attention to and focuses on the importance of particularity and specificity" (Adams, Burke, and Whitmarsh 2014: 182). It recognizes that all knowledge is produced in context and that this context is usually local; it opposes the tendency to push differences in beliefs, practices, and context to the background (Adams, Burke, and Whitmarsh 2014: 181). A strengthened focus on the local does not imply that we analyze specific phenomena in isolation; rather, the local is always connected to a larger context. Taking local realities "on the ground" (Biehl 2007: 107) as a point of departure is important for making "evidence"-based anthropological contributions to the conversation about what works and what needs to change within global health.

This book is based on four related research projects carried out in the same villages. The first project, carried out in 1996 and 1997, focused on health-seeking practices, explanations of illness, and how theories of illness transmission related to spatial practices. During that period, I spent a lot of time in the field getting to know Thomas and his family, who have been among my most important interlocutors. I conducted many interviews with mothers on sickness and childcare, as well as with traditional healers and local experts, many of whom specialized in treating specific symptoms and offered their healthcare services on a part-time basis, spending most of the time tending their fields like any other villager. The second project, carried out in 2001, explored the medical field in more detail, with a specific focus on the use and nonuse of government health facilities. In 2010 and 2011, I revisited Keru, investigating changes within the social and "medical" worlds of the villagers. The third project, which took place from 2012 to 2017,[12] involved a larger research group that examined the relationship between rural citizens and the state. Here, our main purpose was to analyze how rural citizens use government facilities (especially public health care facilities), what rural citizens expect from the state, and how they imagine the state. The project was inspired by the Arab Spring and the unstable political situation in the whole region, where many people forcefully expressed their disappointments with the state. The fourth project, which took place from 2018 to 2023 focused more specifically on state citizen relationship during epidemics with a specific focus on the COVID-19 pandemic. Between these four project periods, I visited the village of Keru on several other occasions as well.

Over the course of two decades, I have conducted hundreds of interviews with villagers in Keru and two neighboring villages, spoken with health care specialists of all kinds, carried out small surveys on treatment-seeking practices, engaged in document research, analyzed health systems reports, and spent hundreds of days observing, conversing, and walking in and between the three villages. The Bancé family has been my anchor throughout my research engagements in Burkina Faso. Each day of fieldwork began by passing by Thomas and Beatrice's compound and saying hello. *Fragile Futures* draws on data from all four projects—and the lives of Thomas, his wife Beatrice, and their seven children play a prominent role in the story. Both Thomas and Beatrice, and Jean, a relative of Thomas I introduce in chapter 1, facilitated my first contacts to many of my interlocutors, and over the years we developed a kind of friendship.[13] They served as gatekeepers (Atkinson 2007) to numerous therapeutic specialists offering their services in the communities. The huge inequalities between the Global North and the Global South become very visible and material during fieldwork like mine, and my long-term engagement with one particular location and with one particular family has generated a number of ethical dilemmas. I have, as many other scholars from the Global North, done my best to be sensitive and to address various ethical challenges.[14] Providing transport to people from the village who needed to go to town and supporting the family and other community members in various ways is of course one way of recognizing otherwise unmet needs. But I am also aware that these small gestures in no way compensate for the obvious and profound inequalities between my life in Denmark and the everyday life of rural citizens in Keru. In addition, I am aware that my presence and my close bonds with the Bancé family most likely also presented them with a range of ethical dilemmas.

One of the goals of this book is to illustrate the continuity and change in Keru and the surrounding villages over two decades. As a result, I am particularly attentive to the temporal context of the specific events or cases I describe. The last chapter of the book is based on data from a new project, Emerging Epidemics: Improving Preparedness in Burkina Faso (2018–2023). The idea for this project arose out of the West African experiences with the Ebola epidemic in 2014 to 2016, long before the COVID-19 outbreak in Wuhan. Due to the worsened security situation, it had become impossible for me to conduct fieldwork in Keru, and due to the COVID-19 outbreak and lockdown, it was not possible to travel to Burkina Faso for a long period. Thus, in this project, I partly relied on remote fieldwork with colleagues living in Bobo-Dioulasso, who managed to conduct interviews on site. Data from this most recent project allows me to examine the state–citizen relationship during a very exceptional period, where the state suddenly emerged as an agent that seemed to care for the people.

The Structure of the Book

The book is organized in three parts dealing with people's active engagement with ambiguities of sickness and care in different types of social relationships: Part I: "Family, Care, and Everyday Life" (chapters 1, 2, and 3); Part II: "Technologies of Care" (chapters 4 and 5); and Part III: "Care of the Public" (chapter 6 and 7).

The first chapter, "A Family Narrative," takes its point of departure from the narrative of the Bancé family. As their experiences demonstrate, village life in Burkina Faso is vibrant, but also tough. It is a life at the margin: contacts with state representatives are rare, and much work is invested in caring for and creating opportunities for the next generation. In this chapter, I introduce the reader to Thomas and Beatrice and their seven children. Thomas, the head of the household, has always been dedicated to being a good citizen: taking responsibility in the village, casting his vote at elections, and encouraging his children to continue schooling and further education. He is a religiously devoted man with high moral standards, but ambiguities concerning how best to care for the family and the future of each of his children are challenging. Following Thomas and Beatrice over more than two decades, I show how they continuously consider options and opportunities in cases of child sickness and reflect carefully about how best to support schooling and job opportunities for each of their seven children, hoping that they will all fare well and be able to support their own families as well as their parents, when Thomas and Beatrice become too old to farm the land.

Chapter 2, "Ambiguities of Child Care," follows up on the story of the sudden death of Caro's small baby. Caro and her in-laws accused each other of causing the death of the child. In this chapter, I show that small children are seen as particularly precarious subjects. During this liminal phase, before another sibling is born, they are both particularly vulnerable and powerful. They are vulnerable in the sense that they can easily die if not properly cared for. They are powerful in the sense that they have a particular relationship with the spiritual world until another sibling is born. This special position is reflected in the ways children are cared for, both when healthy and in times of illness. During early childhood, sickness is part of everyday life (and death): children fall sick, get better, then soon relapse. Child sickness is in this sense endemic rather than episodic. In this chapter, I pay particular attention to the often implicit, unarticulated, and silent care ethics of mothers as the main caregivers (Barnes 2012; Fink 2007; Mol 2008; Van Nistelrooij et al. 2014). The "doing of care" includes hard labor (Arendt 2013; Wilkinson and Kleinman 2016), and seeking treatment is seldom linear. Although consultations at the public health facilities have increased over the years, caregivers continue to juggle between home treatment, consultations with local healing specialists, and visits to the dispensary. By following cases of sickness and listening to mothers' reflections, I demonstrate how families, and mothers in particular, "keep going" in very pragmatic ways, addressing the ambiguities of sickness and care in continuous engagement with uncertainty and hope.

In chapter 3, I focus on labor migration as a form of care work. In the village of Keru most families depend on long-distance social relations, as many young men migrate to other countries to look for work. Many hopes and dreams are invested in the *aventure*,[15] both for those leaving the community and for those staying behind. Labor migration is not only about striving for material gains beyond subsistence agriculture; it is also about care labor, to use Hannah Arendt's distinction between work and labor, and it is about exploring potentialities and taking risks. Michel, the youngest son of Thomas and Beatrice, left for Libya in 2014 to seek work. The story of Michel's *aventure* illustrates the extremely high stakes for the migrants themselves, but also for their families at home. In the second part of this chapter, I focus on the wives whose husbands were away on *aventure*. Among those who "stayed behind," some became even more immobilized, as they were left with all the everyday responsibilities at home. Others managed to find new pathways to generate their own incomes. While many couples had little contact during the often-yearlong migration periods, the husbands remained important "absent-present" figures within the households. Increasing use of mobile phones enabled most wives staying behind to keep contact, at least sporadically, with their absent husbands. However, in their everyday life, these women were engaging with multiple uncertainties, including very concrete uncertainties about how to manage the next meal and the next case of illness, as well as relational uncertainties about their ambiguous position in the household of the absent husband's family. This chapter highlights how labor migration, embarking on *aventure*, presents both the migrant and his or her family staying behind with numerous uncertainties, but also with new opportunities to care for their relatives and to nurse hopes for a good, and perhaps better, future.

In chapter 4, "Technologies and Cosmologies," I focus on care practices in a broader context where various preventive and therapeutic technologies are used to nurse relationships between the individual and society. I argue that certain technologies involve tending relations with the state in order to secure access to public health services while other technologies help cultivate relations with non-human agents in order to confirm connections to the spiritual world. The chapter takes a closer look at the various techniques and technologies used for protection and strengthening of the body. For example, there are similarities between a local incision technique practiced by a local *vaccinatrice* and the biomedical vaccination service provided by the rural health center. While the general utilization of the government health services is relatively low, there is an active demand for vaccinations among rural citizens. Mothers are particular about attending immunization days in order to get their children vaccinated. The chapter also explores the relationship between the popular practice of using amulets to prevent and treat various illnesses and the relatively new practice of using rapid diagnostic tests for malaria at health care facilities. Here the ambiguity of care is not so much about choosing between different preventive or therapeutic logics, but about being open and taking advantage of the available options. By doing so, patients and families of small children confirm both their biosocial citizenship, which authenticates their relationship to the state through signatures of belonging like prescriptions, finger pricks, and vaccination cards, as well as their "spatial citizenship," which reinforces their relationships to the local spiritual world through signatures of belonging such as bodily scars and amulets. Again, tending to relationships both to other people and to non-human agents is important to keep children alive and healthy.

In chapter 5, I describe the therapeutic pathways with a specific focus on how mothers and families navigated between different types of healers and health care institutions. A number of treatment options were available in and around Keru. In addition to the public services, numerous part-time healers and herbal specialists provided services for specific symptoms and diseases. Many ailments were treated at home with herbs collected in the surrounding bush or medicines bought at the local market. I analyze the health care system as a medical field where the different healers and health care institutions position themselves and are positioned through people's therapeutic pathways. The absent-present nature of the public health services places them as just one option among many. For many years, Dr. Sorgho, a relative of Beatrice, was a key figure in the local medical field. As a pensioned government-trained nurse, he had set up a private clinic within his compound where he offered diagnostic and therapeutic services using a biomedical approach. He was extremely popular, and his services competed with the governmental dispensaries in the area. The chapter shows how mothers of sick children seized opportunities for treatment based on their reading of the symptoms, and on their individual constraints and possibilities for maneuvering within the medical field. The high social capital of Dr. Sorgho and many local healing experts also played an important role in local decision-making about whom to consult in case of sickness. The flexible routes between vernacular healing specialists and the public health facilities were saturated with uncertainties and hope, revealing a tension between hoping for something, that is, hoping that each consultation or treatment would result in recovery, and living in hope, that is, reconciling themselves to an everyday life subject to recurrent episodes of sickness (Ricoeur in Huskey 2009). Mothers' therapeutic pathways are undertaken in what Whyte call a *subjunctive mood*, a doubting, hoping, provisional, cautious, and testing disposition to action (Whyte 2005: 250–51).

Chapter 6, "The Availability Logic," explores the services provided at the village dispensary in more detail. In reality, the dispensary was only able to manage a very limited repertoire of diagnoses, so the villagers mainly consulted the dispensary when their sickness corresponded to the diseases the dispensary was able to address. The pattern of diagnosis is a materialization of what I call "the availability logic." A malaria diagnosis was applied in more than half of new clinic visits, and there was a remarkable absence of other presumably frequent diseases. The absence of diagnostic capacity can be seen as a "technology of invisibility" (Biehl 2005), where only a few diseases are named, categorized, and reported. In line with discussions of the importance of statistics (Adams 2016; Wendland 2016), I raise questions about the consequences of having a routinized—and almost ritualized—consultation practice, where many ailments remain invisible and unreported, either because they are never brought to the dispensary or because the diagnostic capacity at the facility is limited. The social contract between the government's health care services and rural citizens remained weak throughout my study of health-seeking processes in Keru. Despite a number of improvements over the years, including the use of rapid diagnostic tests, the duties of the modern state to care for the health of its citizens, as embedded in the term "public health" (Prince and Marsland 2014), were never really followed through.

In chapter 7, "Moments of State Presence," the focus of attention shifts from the routines of the dispensary in Keru to state–citizen dynamics during the COVID-19 pandemic in 2020 and 2021. Based on public announcements, readings of plans and policies, and a series of conversations with urban citizens in Bobo-Dioulasso, the second largest city in Burkina Faso, I discuss how local responses to the epidemic and the precautionary measures introduced by the government temporarily affected and changed relationships between citizens and the state. Despite the relatively mild course of the epidemic in the country in terms of registered cases and COVID-related deaths, COVID-19 was talked about as an exceptional disease, as an epidemic like no previous epidemics. I argue here that the exceptionality of COVID-19 compared to previous epidemics was not so much related to its specific risks or symptoms, but rather to the fact that people had never before experienced a government that introduced such severe general restrictions in order to safeguard the health of the population. The otherwise "absent" or distant government had suddenly stepped in and deployed its sovereign authority and biopower to "discipline the population" in order to preempt an uncertain future of COVID-19 in Burkina Faso. In this specific situation, the state responded to the wish that it care for its citizens, although some critique remained.

In the conclusion, I briefly summarize my main arguments with an emphasis on rural citizens' openness to different interpretations and their continuous work with potentialities and hope in a social, political, and economic context shaped by global inequalities and specific regional and national insecurities. Over time, improvements in public health care services have materialized: a new dispensary was built in Keru (now equipped with electricity), the rapid diagnostic test for malaria became a routine, and after 2016, free health care for children under five was introduced. The number of consultations at public biomedical health facilities has increased over the years, yet rural citizens continue to explore and juggle between different treatment options, including self-treatment at home and consultations with vernacular healing experts. This is not only due to a lack of diagnostic technologies and qualified staff at the public health facilities; citizens are actors with pragmatic and open minds trying to alleviate suffering and manage the ambiguities of sickness through engaged social encounters with different types of experts. The relationship between citizens and the state remains in many ways weak; still, the state is present in people's perceptions, engagements, and hopes for a better future as observed during the COVID-19 pandemic, where many people praised (at least temporarily) the government for deploying statecraft and willingness to care for ordinary people. Lastly, I discuss future perspectives for health care in Burkina Faso and reflect on how this ethnography of the social imaginaries of health care and health care institutions may contribute to a more general discussion of health care systems in the Global South.

Notes

1. Village names and the names of my interlocutors are all pseudonyms.
2. I call her Caro from this point.
3. The Fragile States Index (formerly known as the Failed States Index), developed by the US think tank Fund for Peace together with the magazine *Foreign Policy*, is published annually. All sovereign states that are members of the United Nations are assessed in terms of their vulnerability to conflict or collapse. Fragile States Index, "Country Dashboard." Retrieved 10 October 2020 from https://fragilestatesindex.org/country-data/.
4. Fragile States Index, "P2: Public Services." Retrieved 13 May 2021 from https://fragilestatesindex.org/indicators/p2/.
5. Recently, the use of *fragile state* as a specific term has been critiqued for simplifying complex situations and underpinning the notion that international interventions are necessary to mitigate the risks they pose. Danish Institute

for International Studies, "Fragile States" policy brief, 9 March 2022. Retrieved 13 July 2023 from https://www.diis.dk/en/research/fragile-states.

6. UNDP, "Burkina Faso," Human Development Report 2020. Retrieved 17 August 2023 from https://hdr.undp.org/data-center/specific-country-data#/countries/BFA
7. In 2019, Burkina Faso ranked 182 out of 189 countries. UNDP, *Human Development Reports*. Retrieved 17 August from https://hdr.undp.org/content/human-development-report-2019
8. Macrotrends. Retrieved 02 October, 2023 from https://www.macrotrends.net/countries/BFA/burkina-faso/population-growth-rate.
9. United Nations, *A Survey on Migration Policies in West Africa*, ch. on Burkina Faso. Retrieved 13 July 2023 from https://www.un.org/development/desa/pd/sites/www.un.org.development.desa.pd/files/unpd_ws_201509_burkina faso_migration_fact_sheet.pdf
10. Just as the pilots' vomit, sweat, and fear do not fit into the aircraft brochures (Law 2002: 98).
11. The traditional chieftain system is not part of the official state apparatus, but the chiefs are recognized by the government and play important roles in conflict management at the village level (Cissao 2020).
12. The 1996–1997 project was generously funded by the Danish Bilharziasis Laboratory and was undertaken as part of my PhD in Anthropology at the University of Copenhagen, Denmark. The 2001 study was funded by the Council for Development Research under Danida (RUF journal no. 91092). The 2010 study was funded by the Carlsberg Foundation and included two terms as by-fellow at Churchill College, University of Cambridge, UK (project no. 2009_01_063). The 2012–2017 study was funded by the Ministry of Foreign Affairs of Denmark (Danida project no. 11–014-KU). Chapter 7 is mainly based on a collaborative project entitled Emerging Epidemics: Improving Preparedness in Burkina Faso, funded by the Ministry of Foreign Affairs (Danida project no 17–06-KU). My field trips to Burkina Faso after 2018 were financed by this project. Research permission has been granted by CNRST (Centre National de Recherche Scientifique et Technologique) in Burkina Faso.
13. I agree with Michael Jackson that "there is often a world of difference between these bonds of kinship and friendship in the field, and nominally identical bonds back home. The intimate and incorporative bonds of fictive kinships and friendships that belong to the fieldwork situation are frequently opportunistic and transitory, what they often connote is a deep sense of gratitude that the ethnographer feels toward his host community for having saved his or her sense of dignity in a culturally disorientating and debilitating environment" (1998: 104). While my relationships with Thomas, Beatrice, Jean, and others may have included opportunistic elements, they have not been transitory. Even though traveling to Burkina Faso has been restricted over the last couple of years due to the COVID-19 pandemic and the tense security situation in the country, I continue to stay in contact with family members via WhatsApp.

14. All the research projects involving fieldwork have received the necessary research permissions and ethical clearance.
15. As Jesper Bjarnesen highlights (2013: 24), labor migration represents an important sociocultural process in the lives of the migrants and their families in Burkina Faso: "The move away from home is often inscribed into local cosmologies as a move towards maturity and independence." The word *aventure* (adventure) alludes to the double perspective of a journey full of uncertainties but also with openings and potentials.

Part I

Family, Care, and Everyday Life

Chapter 1
A Family Narrative

Like most other residents in Keru, Thomas spent much of his time tending his fields—some of which were located close to the village, others were situated more than twenty kilometers away. It is difficult to be a farmer in Burkina Faso. A successful harvest depends on one rainy season, from May to September or October, with huge fluctuations from year to year. Some years the rain may fall in short, intense periods, making it impossible for the soil to absorb it; other years the rain is sparse, resulting in a poor harvest. The fact that a whole year's supply of maize, millet, and sorghum depends on one rather unpredictable rainy season makes the livelihood of the local farmers fragile. Just before the harvest, everything looks luxuriant, with crops standing high (at least in the "good" years), while after the harvest everything becomes dry and sandy until the next growing season.

Almost half the population in Burkina Faso lives below the poverty line of US$1.90 per day, and poverty rates in rural areas are almost three times those of urban areas (UNDP 2019). For the 70 to 80 percent of Burkina's population living in rural areas, including those in Keru and the neighboring villages (Faure 1990; Samuelsen 1999), subsistence agriculture is the main economic activity (Belesova et al. 2019), though it is supported by (irregular) remittances from family members working at farms or mines in other regions of Burkina Faso or in neighboring countries (Ajefu and Ogebe 2021; Wouterse 2010). Most of the agricultural products are consumed by households themselves, while a smaller part is sold at the local market. The main crops are millet, sorghum, maize, groundnuts, white beans, peas, and rice. Cotton and tobacco are also grown as cash crops in this area but to a lesser extent. Vegetable gardens, with tomatoes, onions, eggplants, lettuce, and carrots, are mainly organized by women's groups (Groupement Villagois). The staple food in this part of the country is *tô*, a porridge made of millet or maize. Red sorghum is mainly used for beer production (Sarrassat et al. 2019), which plays a significant role in the local economy, particularly for the female beer producers, known as *dolotières*. On low-lying land (the *bas-fonds*), the villagers grow rice wherever possible.

In this chapter, I paint a picture of the everyday life of Thomas and his family. Their story, and the story of others in Keru, tells a good deal about the hardships, challenges, hopes, and aspirations facing those in rural Burkina Faso. I hope to show how health, illness, the economy, and political changes have affected the people of rural Africa over the past twenty-five years. The experience of Thomas and his family likely resembles that of many other families living in low-income societies. As João Biehl and Adriana Petryna put it:

> These peopled accounts—stories that are so often hidden from view, obscured by more abstract and bureaucratic considerations of public policy—are the very fabric of alternative social theorizing. By looking closely at life stories and at the ups and downs of individuals and communities as they grapple with inequality, struggle to access technology, and confront novel state-market formations, we begin to apprehend larger systems. We are able to see them in the making or in the process of dissolution, and we understand more intimately the local realities, so often unspoken, that result when people are seen or governed in a particular way, or not at all. (Biehl and Petryna 2013: 2–3)

The village of Keru is located at the margins of the state in more than one sense. It is geographically far from the political elites, important business communities, and key governmental institutions. The infrastructure "thins out" as the distance from the urban areas increases, and the few government institutions in rural areas are under-resourced, offering poor-quality services. The spatial margins are political, social, and economic as well. In line with Biehl and Petryna (2013) and Dorothy Hodgson (2017), I argue that stories from the margins, such as the stories about Thomas and his family, offer key theoretical and political insights into larger structural issues and highlight local, often unspoken realities. They also bear witness to a vibrant agency among rural residents and portray how people secure a safe future for themselves and their families through a strong critical awareness about what to expect and what not to expect from the ruling elite. In other words, such stories "defy enduring stereotypes about the passivity and ignorance of rural peoples," as Hodgson (2017: 38) notes. Furthermore, by taking the perspectives of a rural village and one particular family as my point of departure, I hope to illustrate that marginality goes both ways: not only is the village marginal for the state, but the state, through its elusive character and its many absences, was in some ways also marginal to the everyday life of rural citizens in Keru.

In daily life, there is a lot of movement in and out of Keru. During the rainy season (when the sowing takes place) and during the harvest, the level of activity is particularly high, with both men and women passing to and from their fields, many of which are located far away from the village. During these periods, it is hard to find any adults at home during the day. In addition, the village members spend their time collecting firewood for cooking, gathering leaves for various sauces accompanying *tô*, and picking items to use in the preparation of various items to sell, such as shea butter and herbal medicine. In addition, barks, leaves, roots, and herbs are often collected for medical purposes (Samuelsen 1999: 20–25; 2004b).

Keru is a patrilineal and virilocal society. The Bancé family is exogamous; they marry outside the village, and sons cannot marry close relatives on their mother's side. The local farmers do not have private ownership of their land, as most land in rural Burkina Faso is owned by the state and administered under community customary law (Bambio and Agha 2018). Land use is inherited from father to son, and the land cannot be bought or sold. Thomas and his brother inherited their land from their father, and Thomas's two sons will probably take over from him, dividing the land between them, or, if they agree, having one of them continue the farming activities while the other finds a job outside the village. Upon marriage, the husband may allocate a piece of land for his wife to tend.

When I started fieldwork in 1996, most houses in Keru were small, round mud houses with thatched roofs. Each adult had his or her own house. Small children and older girls slept in their mother's house while boys, after reaching a certain age, slept together in a separate house. Most people did not have any furniture inside their houses; they slept on plastic mats, which they rolled out at night, either inside the house or, during the dry season, outside in the courtyard. The women often kept some of their harvest in jars or sacks, and their personal belongings such as clothes and pots were either kept in a metal box or stored in a sack inside their houses (Fainzang 1986; Samuelsen 1999). A mud wall with one main entrance encircled each family homestead. In compounds with extended families, lower walls inside the compound served to separate the households—each consisting of a man, his wife or wives, and children—from each other. Most compounds had a shelter (*hangar*) made of branches and hay either inside the compound or just outside. Household members would often sit under the shelter working at various household chores or use it as a shady place for entertaining guests. The compounds did not include latrines, but often a wall inside the compound designated a small place reserved for washing and urinating. Over the years, it has become much more common to construct square cement houses with corrugated tin roofs. Such houses are more solidly built compared to the traditional mud and clay houses, and they are more suitable for the heavy seasonal rains. Building a new house back home is the first priority for migrants, and they often earmark remittances for this purpose, gradually building a home as their income allows. Thomas had been able to save money to construct two new houses within his compound, a small house for himself and a large two-room house for his wife and their daughters. Recently, Pascal, their eldest son, had also constructed a small square house with a corrugated roof inside the family compound for himself. He had been away briefly as a migrant worker but had to return home because of an injury. In chapter 3, I will return to the migrant experiences of Thomas's two sons.

Keru means "place of happiness." The Bancé family, to which Thomas belongs, was said to be the founding family of the village and was still one of the dominant families in the village; in fact, the traditional chief was a member of the family. According to the elders in the village, Keru had been established as a village before the area was colonized. From 1884 to 1890, French, English, and German colonizers tried to include this region as part of their colonial territory (Faure 1996: 99–103). It became part of the French West African colony called French Sudan, but the borders of the colony changed over time. From 1902 to 1904, the region was part of Territoire de la Sénégambie-Niger; from 1904 to 1919, it was part of Haut Sénégal-Niger; and from 1919 to 1933, it was called Terri-

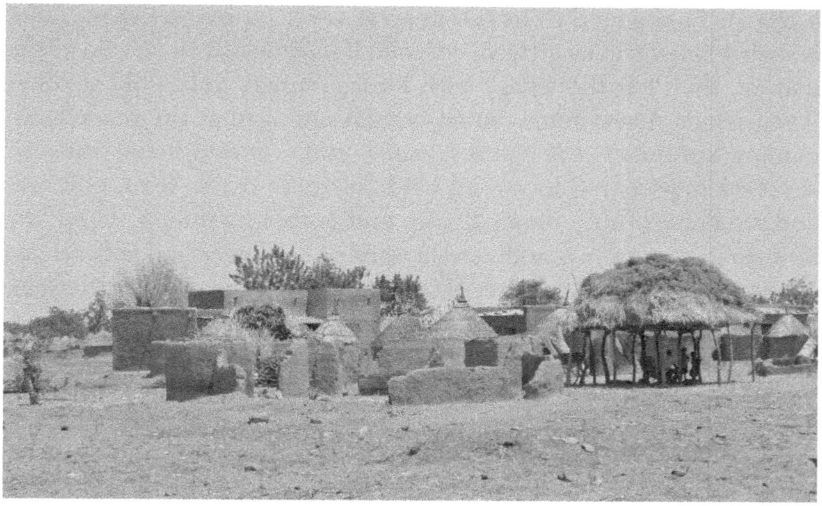

Figure 1.1. Rural household, Burkina Faso (© Helle Samuelsen 2023)

toire de la Haute Volta. After 1933, it was united with Côte d'Ivoire, then from 1947 to 1960 it was reconstituted as Haute Volta, with the same borders as in the period from 1919 to 1933 (Lahuec and Marchal 1979). Burkina Faso became independent in 1960, as did many other African states. The traditional system with local chiefs continues to coexist with the formal political system. The local chief of Keru was a relatively well-off man who owned a substantial number of cattle and was involved in various small-scale businesses, in addition to his farming activities. He was a very friendly man who lived in a huge compound in the central part of the village. Many of his sons and male family members had migrated to neighboring countries for work, and a few had even migrated to Italy.[1] At a visit in 2013, he told me that his household "normally" would include around 180 people, but since many family members had migrated, "only" 109 were left.

Keru is a fairly large village with 1,757 inhabitants in 1998 and 2,383 in 2006.[2] It is well-known in the region for its large market located in the village center. There are a few permanent shops, bicycle and motorcycle workshops, restaurants, and tailors, but on market days the whole place is buzzing with all types of traders, who find shade under a few old trees and a number of shelters. Over the years, the market has grown significantly. At the beginning of my fieldwork, a few pickups came from the nearest town on market days; later, heavily loaded trucks arrived with all kinds of goods to be sold at the market, then left the village with local products to be sold at other destinations. Everything can be bought and sold at the market, including European-style clothes, *pagne* (cloth for traditional dresses), vegetables, prepared foods, all kinds of spare parts, soap, chicken, and medicines (both biomedicines and herbal products). There are also small restaurants and taverns serving cold beer and soft drinks. Market day takes place every third day in Keru throughout the year, attracting people from many of the neighboring villages. In 2018, electricity was installed in the village. While individual households do not have electrical connections, the shops and taverns at the market are now connected. A bustling cattle and goat market, which is open on the same days as the central market, is located at the border of the village. The buying and selling of animals is mainly a business activity for men, while vegetable and fruit sales are primarily carried out by women.

Thomas

Thomas told me about his troubles with a thrombosis in his right leg when we met early one afternoon at a local restaurant in Dassasgo, a suburb of Ouagadougou, in 2019. Late one evening a few months earlier, while he was in bed, he felt an immense pain that kept him awake. Thomas sleeps in his own small one-room house, while his wife Beatrice and the other female members of the household sleep in another small house within the same compound. As his pain worsened, he was afraid that he would pass away. At five in the morning, he decided to wake up Pascal, his eldest son, who slept in his own room near the entrance of the compound, and he asked Pascal to take him to the dispensary. Pascal accompanied him to the clinic, where they knocked on the door and woke up the nurse. The nurse found that Thomas's blood pressure was much too high and that his right leg was almost paralyzed. He was then admitted to the dispensary for observation and given medication to lower his blood pressure. In the following months, he visited the local dispensary every two weeks for checkups and took his medicine every morning and evening. He explained: "I go to the dispensary for my checkups and I pay 200 CFA [franc]. Now it is OK. They prescribe the medicines. If

I have the money, I buy the medicines; if I don't have money, I wait until I have money and then I buy the medicines." In addition to the medication, the nurse advised him to massage his leg every day with an ointment. Despite the treatment, his sense of balance was weakened, and he had trouble walking, which made working in the fields more difficult.

I first met Thomas through contacts in Ouagadougou as I was searching for a rural fieldwork location in Burkina Faso for my doctoral project. My contact in Ouagadougou was related to Thomas and suggested that I ask him to be my interpreter in the field. I was introduced to Thomas at my very first visit to Keru. He was one of the residents who assisted us when our car got stuck in the mud. We had turned off the main road onto the long dirt road to the village. The late-summer rainy season was at its peak, and the twenty-kilometer drive was difficult to traverse even with four-wheel drive. Thomas welcomed us to the village with a warm and friendly smile. I was happy to be so kindly received and immediately felt at ease. Since my first day in the field, Thomas's great hospitality has been of tremendous value both for me and my family and for the students I brought with me to the field. Eventually, Thomas became one of my key interlocutors and gatekeepers, and our friendship developed over the years.

When we met at the restaurant in Dassasgo, Thomas was dressed in a long shirt with printed religious motifs, the sleeves decorated with laces, and a pair of loose trousers in a similar print. It was a type of clothing he often wore when participating in public and religious activities outside his home. A necklace with a cross proclaimed his affiliation to the Catholic Church—for many years he had served as the local catechist in Keru. A small knitted cap covered his short gray hair. That afternoon, as on so many previous occasions, Thomas and I started our conversation by exchanging the latest news from our families and about everyday life in Keru; this time we also talked a lot about the increasingly tense political and security situation in the country.

The escalating terrorism in Burkina Faso had led to numerous travel restrictions for foreigners, so it had not been possible for me to travel to Keru to conduct fieldwork in the same way as I had done so many times before. According to the security map developed by the French Ministry of Foreign Affairs, all border areas to Mali, Niger, Benin, and Togo, as well as fourteen districts within Burkina Faso, were formally designated "red zones," where travel was not recommended, and the rest of the country was categorized as "orange zones," where travel was not recommended unless one had specific reasons. The Danish embassy in Ouagadougou had advised me not to make any trips outside the capital, as terrorist attacks against foreigners and against representatives of nongovernmental organizations (NGOs) and the government were occurring more and more frequently. Because of this, I had invited Thomas to Ouagadougou so we could talk in person. When I first suggested, during a telephone conversation, that he could come to the capital to see me, he sounded puzzled. Had it really become that dangerous to move around in Burkina Faso? Although he was fully updated about the various terrorist attacks inside Burkina Faso, village life continued as usual. When I explained that the Danish embassy had strongly advised against moving outside of the capital, he immediately agreed to the plan and decided to use the opportunity to visit relatives living in the city while he was there.

At the age of sixty-five, Thomas continued to be a very energetic man, but age was beginning to affect his everyday life. He was still head of the family and still active in farming the fields he owned outside his natal village of Keru. Like many other people in their sixties who had labored for many years in the fields, Thomas suffered from arthritis. In addition, some years back he had undergone cataract surgery in both eyes. Besides these age-related conditions and recurring episodes of seasonal malaria throughout his life, Thomas had been in good health. That afternoon, sitting comfortably at the local restaurant sharing a Coke and a beer, he was in good spirits, exhibiting his usual combination of seriousness, especially when talking about his seven children and the development of the country, and humor. Thomas had always been easy to talk with, although he often became more formal when we met in places other than his family compound, where most of our conversations over the years had taken place. Although the atmosphere was casual, finding a good time and the best place to meet had taken several telephone conversations. The restaurant we chose was located in a spacious garden. Rusty metal tables and chairs had been placed on the sandy ground with a few trees and bushes providing a little shade for the guests. It was a discreet place where we could talk quietly; besides the waiter who served us more Cokes and beers, and eventually a meal, we were not disturbed.

Thomas had lived in Keru all his life, except for three years when he was a catechist in the neighboring village of Tenga. As a member of one of the founding families of the village and a faithful participant in the region's Catholic mission, Thomas seemed to be a cherished community member. He had no formal positions in the village nor was he well-off, but he was highly respected. Fellow villagers often consulted him in matters of personal crisis and family conflict. He worked hard to live up to his own expectations of being a good citizen: he sent all seven children to school, he took responsibility in the village, he prioritized his scarce resources, and he acted swiftly in cases of sickness. It had not always been easy. He was a religiously devoted man with a strong ethos and high moral standards, but he was challenged by environmental and socioeconomic conditions as well as by his own family. In the following chapters, I return to specific cases and narratives of individual members of Thomas's family. Here, I introduce them and their everyday life in more detail.

Thomas's family belongs to the Bissa, a relatively small ethnic group that makes up 3.7 percent of Burkina's population.[3] Originally, all Bissa people spoke Bissa, but today most people in Keru speak Mooré, the language of the Mossi, the country's largest ethnic group (52 percent of the population).[4] The Bissa-speaking residents are primarily women who never attended school. Thomas spoke French and Mooré, but he did not speak Bissa fluently, although he understood it. His wife Beatrice spoke Bissa and Mooré fluently, but very little French. The Bissa region is located in the central-east part of Burkina, and Tenkodogo, Garango, and Zabré are its largest towns. The population in this area is ethnically mixed, with people from the Bissa, Mossi, Yarsi, and Peuhl ethnic groups. According to Armelle Faure (1996), a village is defined as a Bissa village in this region if the *chef de village* (the village chief) defines himself as Bissa. This was the case in Keru, but, as we shall see later, the ethnic identity of villages in this area was a controversial issue. Before (and to a certain extent after) colonization, this area had been dominated by the highly centralized Mossi kingdom, with less centralized ethnic groups, including the Bissa, in the periphery. Tensions between Bissa residents and the Mossi kingdom had existed both before and after independence in 1960, as Bissa people often protested against the requirement to pay taxes to the Mossi king. On the first day of my very first visit to the area, my Bissa contact in Ouagadougou advised me to pay a courtesy visit to the *Samadin*, the "foreign minister" of the *Mogho Naba*, the Mossi king, to get approval from the head of the traditional chiefs to conduct fieldwork in their area. Ethnic conflicts between the Mossi and the Bissa had grown over the last decades—there were a few violent incidents and a number of court cases over land-use rights—although intermarriage between Bissa and Mossi families was common. More recently, a number of Bissa-dominated villages had elected their own Bissa chief in an effort to replace the "traditional" Mossi chief approved by the Mossi king, with the result that some villages had two chiefs, one Bissa and one Mossi (Cissao 2019).

Beatrice

Beatrice, Thomas's wife, organized her *cabaret* (home-based millet beer tavern) every three days all year-round to coincide with the market days. The traditional preparation of *dolo* (millet beer) involves several steps, including malting the red sorghum grains followed by crushing, mashing, cooking, lactic acid fermenting, filtering, boiling, and alcoholic fermenting (Pale et al. 2010; Saul 1981). It is a labor-intensive activity. A large amount of water has to be fetched from the village water pump, and enough firewood has to be collected for four hours of boiling on the first day and eight to nine hours of boiling on the second day. A small portion of the beer may be consumed unfermented before the addition of the yeast on the second night. On the third morning, the *dolo* is poured into small jars, ready to be sold. *Dolo* is a brownish-red cloudy drink with a sweet and sour taste containing up to 5 percent alcohol by volume. At Beatrice's cabaret, the *dolo* was usually served in a small calabash at a cost of 50 CFA (US$0.10). This was a relatively good business for her. As in many other parts of Africa, husbands and wives have separate finances, so Beatrice kept the income from the *cabaret* to herself (spending most of it on food and clothes for their children). She also had to buy the sorghum, either from Thomas or from other sorghum producers in the village. Beatrice's daughters helped her with the beer production, and for several years all the hard work was carried out by the eldest daughter living at home—first Sylvie, and then the others: Myriel, Caroline,[5] and eventually the two youngest, Janine and Claudine, who had less and less time to help their mother prepare the millet beer because they were busy with school. Beatrice made high-quality *dolo* that tasted good, which was recognized by the many people in Keru who regularly turned up for a drink. Although *dolo* is not a strong beverage, people who stopped by the cabaret often drank a lot, and it was not unusual to hear and see a few drunk men and women there in the late afternoon. Beatrice appreciated her many customers as well as the social life her *cabaret* generated. Over the course of time, her own intake of *dolo* had increased, sometimes to an extent that I sensed Thomas found inappropriate. The *cabarets* had a very important social role in the village, and although most Muslims do not drink alcohol, it was not unusual to see both Christians and Muslims at the local *cabarets*. Sometimes, a *griot* (Kaschula 1999) passed by, and these older men often received a calabash of *dolo* for free while telling a story or playing a tune on a simple string instrument or on small drums. With the high temperatures that prevail almost year-round in this part of Africa, *dolo* is also simply a liquid that quenches one's thirst, particularly when drinking water is available only at a few pumps in the village.

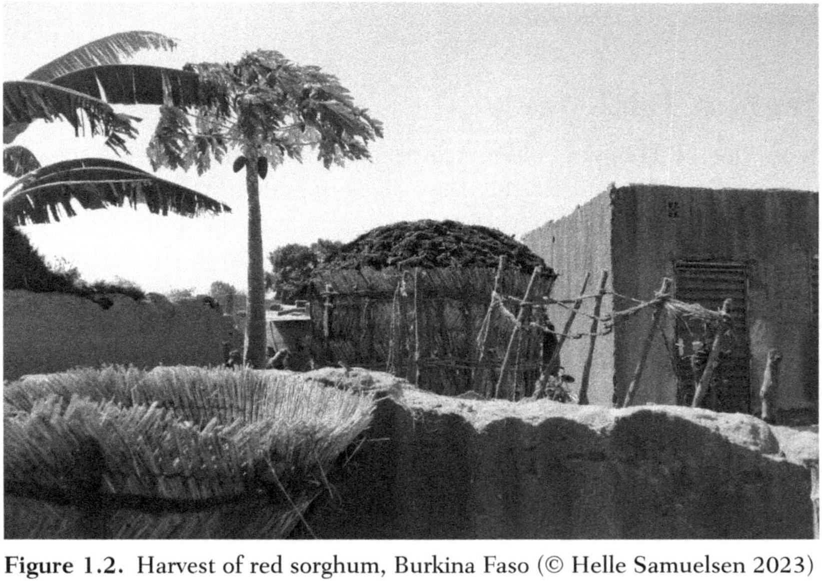

Figure 1.2. Harvest of red sorghum, Burkina Faso (© Helle Samuelsen 2023)

Beatrice was a devoted Catholic and active in the local church, although her own family was Muslim. She converted to Christianity just before marrying Thomas and changed her name from Binta to Beatrice. She often wore *pagne* (the traditional dress), which consists of a large piece of printed cloth wrapped around the waist as a skirt with a smaller piece of cloth in a similar design covering her hair. When dressing up, many women wear a small blouse made of the same fabric and a length of cloth with a similar print to carry a small child on their back. In everyday life, many women wear a T-shirt with the *pagne*. For religious rituals or festivals, Thomas and Beatrice had outfits made with identical prints and religious motifs. Beatrice was a very independent woman with her own opinions. It was my impression that they discussed many issues jointly as a couple, particularly concerning the future plans of their children. Both encouraged their children to continue schooling, and Beatrice was proud of how well her two youngest daughters had done in school. She was also very concerned about the family economy. During my first period of fieldwork, when we discussed the possibility of Thomas being my interpreter, Beatrice suggested a salary double what Thomas suggested, and during her daughter Janine's time at university, Beatrice asked her to explain all of her expenses in order to ensure that Janine economized the support she received from home.

Jean, a Trickster

Jean, one of Thomas's older relatives, guided and facilitated my understanding of medicine that took place outside of the formal health care system. He had a vast knowledge about the local flora and about medicinal use of bark, leaves, and roots from the bush areas around Keru. He also had a wide network—everybody seemed to know him. This also included the many local healers, who often saw their knowledge and skills as a privilege that should be guarded. Jean explained to them the purpose of my study and my interest in their healing skills, and he also exchanged some of his own experiences with them. As a result, they were all willing to explain their practices to us, although I am sure they also kept some secrets to themselves. Jean and I conducted many interviews and conversations with herbal specialists, marabouts (Qur'an specialists), diviners, and so-called charlatans, and we had several conversations with the only sorcery specialist in the village. When I showed Jean the book *Trees and Shrubs of the Sahel* (von Maydell 1986), he participated enthusiastically in identifying the Latin names of the plants used by the various healers.

Jean had a trickster-like position in the local community. Although the trickster figure appears mainly in myths and tales (Babcock-Abrahams 1975; Levi-Strauss 1963; Pelton 1989), Jean's role in Keru shared some similar characteristics.[6] The classic trickster figures are from the tales of North American native groups and gain their power from their embodiment of opposing propensities (Levi-Strauss 1963). The fundamental trait of the trickster is ambiguity, though the trickster also has related identities as a trick-player, a shape shifter, a situation-inverter, a messenger of the gods, and a sacred/lewd bricoleur (Hynes 1993). Although Jean was a member of the village's founding family, his status was ambiguous. Like Legba in the West African myth, he was both a troublemaker and someone who could bring order through rituals (Sjørslev 2015: 131). Jean sometimes discussed matters in a loud voice, and he loved to provoke, but he was also very serious and reflective. While Thomas often tried to downplay or "talk around" some of the so-called traditional treatment practices that did not correspond with the Christian faith, Jean was very open about all types of medical and religious practices. It was Jean who introduced me, without hesitation, to the sorcery specialist and to the diviner.

Jean lived for many years alone in a small, dilapidated house rather than in a family compound. It is very unusual for a man to live alone in rural Burkina Faso—it was some months into my time in Burkina Faso before he told me about his marriage, explaining that his wife and children lived with her parents in a household in another section of the village. His wife was affected mentally after a meningitis infection during her childhood. She was unable to cook for herself and her family, but she helped with many practical chores in her parents' household. They had four children who lived with their mother and grandparents throughout their childhood.

Jean was a small skinny man with only two or three teeth, and he was always wearing dirty and worn-out clothes and a pair of white plastic sandals with broken straps. However, he was smart and full of energy, always ready with a quick joke, often a dirty one, when passing community members in the village. Jean was poor, and he often tried to get snacks and *dolo* for free, but he was nevertheless a very respected person and able to transgress all kinds of boundaries. He was in his late forties when I first met him, and was the only man of his generation that I ever saw playing soccer with the boys in the village. He was Christian and active in the church, but he lived in a predominantly Muslim quarter of the village. He did not have a formal role within the Catholic community, but he sat in the corner of the local church with drummers and singers, playing the rattle. He also had a privileged relationship to several marabouts, diviners, and local herbalists. He had been the village representative when the government of Burkina Faso, in collaboration with the Danish development organization DANIDA, installed water pumps in the village, and he became the person responsible for the maintenance of the pumps, entrusted with the key to lock and unlock them. For some years, he also worked as a "bureaucrat," collecting taxes at the cow, sheep, and goat market. For each transaction, a small fee had to be paid to the municipality, and it was Jean's job to collect these fees. On market days, I often saw him walking resolutely toward the marketplace with a thin briefcase under his arm, though I am not sure how systematic this tax collection really was.

One year during my first period of fieldwork, Jean also took on a very different role. He was asked to be responsible for the yearly village *tenkande* (sacrifice) ritual in which sacrifices are made to the earth on behalf of the eldest villagers. The *tenkande* is performed at an open spot near the marketplace where the village altar (a set of three stones) is located. The sacrifice is performed by male members of the community to make a collective wish for a good harvest, but individual people, both men and women, are allowed to sacrifice for their own future prosperity and that of their family. I was allowed to participate in one such ritual.

Starting very early in the morning, the village elders, the four or five oldest members of the community, sat in a circle around the altar. Many community members, mainly males, joined the ceremony and sat in wider circles. That year, Jean performed the ritual on behalf of the elders because the oldest man in the village felt too weak to perform it himself. A young man handed the objects to be sacrificed to Jean. First, sacrifices were made on behalf of the whole village; each quarter of the village was represented, and general wishes for the future of the village were expressed. Jean was sitting just next to the altar stones, stripped to the waist. With a solemn expression, he called on the ancestors and on God, performing the sacrifices on behalf of the community as a whole and on behalf of individual members. Blood from chickens, eggs, *tô*, *dolo* and water, chicken and goat meat, galettes (small locally produced flat cakes), pieces of goatskin and sheepskin, and money were smashed at the altar stones as part of the sacrifice. The atmosphere was intense. People contributed money of various amounts, coins of 25 CFA were collected in a bowl, and larger pieces of meat were donated and placed near Jean, who left some of the bones at the altar. The good pieces of meat were later distributed among the various families represented at the event; Jean was in charge of the redistribution with the help of two young men who had cut up the meat in smaller pieces (Samuelsen 1999: 106–110). Jean and the other elders expressed their wishes for a profitable next harvest and for the village's health and prosperity.

Suddenly, an old man shouted loudly. He looked angry and smashed an egg hard on the altar stones. It turned out that someone had recently stolen a sheep and a guinea fowl from him, and by doing a sacrifice, he hoped that the thief would soon be caught. Then, individuals went up to Jean and gave him items, such as chickens, *dolo*, or eggs that they wished to sacrifice individually. He made the sacrifice on the altar stones, and people expressed their wishes for the future or thanked God and their ancestors for good events of the past. A young man sacrificed a cock and a piece of goat meat, wishing he would find a good woman to marry in the coming year. A woman also sacrificed a piece of goat meat, thanking the supreme powers for listening to her previous wishes for more children. At the time of her previous sacrifice, she had only one child; now she had four children, and she wanted to give thanks for this prosperity. Another woman made a sacrifice because she was childless and wanted children. A young man made a sacrifice with the desire to earn lots of money and promised that he would sacrifice a whole sheep the following year if he succeeded in becoming rich.

Jean spoke loudly and clearly, and all the participants watched and listened attentively, but as the morning progressed, the atmosphere became more relaxed. Some people left and others arrived. Many children were crowding around the altar stones to get a good look; a few of them were reprimanded when they moved too close. According to Faure (1996), who described the *tenkande* ritual of another Bissa village, Ouarègou, the prayers are meant to address Woso (God), Tara (the domesticated land), and Toor (the territorial spirits). In Keru, the sacrifices were primarily directed toward Wende (God) and the ancestors. All quarters of the village were represented at the ritual, which, as the village chief explained, "recognizes the history and culture of the village."

Jean died of a heart attack in 2005. I had been away from the village for a long period and only heard about his death when I came back in 2010. He had suffered from heart problems for several years. During my first period in the field, I had been to the village on a Friday to do some interviews, and when I passed by Jean's compound to say hello, he was lying inside his house, not feeling well. He came out and talked for a few minutes. He did not look well, but it was difficult to say how serious his illness was. However, a few days later, he told me that he had almost died. His heart had stopped beating, "mais Dieu est grand" (but God is great), as he said, and he quickly recovered. Thomas confirmed that it had been a serious incident and told me that he had stopped by to check up on Jean after I had left the village.

The Children

I arrived in Keru on election day in November 2015, having visited a couple of polling places along the dirt road from the provincial town. It was market day in Keru, and Beatrice's *cabaret* was full of people in high spirits. Beatrice jumped up as soon as she saw me entering the compound, then hugged me and kissed me on the cheeks, as the French do. She was in a good mood, as were the other guests at her *cabaret*, and she did a few dance steps to welcome me. Sylvie, the eldest daughter, shouted excitedly and came over to me, lifting me up and giving me a big hug. Feeling happy about the warm welcome, I also realized that this election day was a very special day for the citizens of Keru, a day worth celebrating. Thomas invited me to the inner courtyard, where I was seated in one of the old white metal chairs in the shade under a small shelter. Sitting here with a small calabash of Beatrice's refreshing *dolo*, I heard the latest news about Thomas and Beatrice's seven children.

Pascal, the oldest child, now thirty-six years old, was helping Thomas to farm the fields, and during afternoons and on market days, he sold soft drinks and bottled beer at his small *buvette* in the marketplace. Some years back, he had tried his luck as a migrant worker in Côte d'Ivoire. This *aventure*, as migrant work is called in most parts of West Africa, had however not been successful. He had injured his left leg in an accident, which had left him with a large unhealed wound. This injury continued to cause him trouble many years later. He had therefore returned home and was now living in his parental home, still unmarried. Pascal's story is in no way exceptional. Many young men from Keru and other villages in the region who migrate do not succeed in earning a stable income that allows them to support their families at home (Kleist and Bjarnesen 2019).

Thomas and Beatrice's younger son, Michel, was not at home. He had left for Libya in 2014. I was in Burkina Faso that year as the family discussed the possibility that he would migrate. Originally, they had decided that he should go to Guinea or Côte d'Ivoire as many other young men from the village had, but at the time of his departure, the southern border of Burkina Faso was closed because of the Ebola epidemic in Sierra Leone, Guinea, and Liberia. After consultation with the family, Michel decided to try his luck in the north, traveling through the Sahara Desert to search for work in Libya. In chapter 3, I unfold the migration stories of Pascal and Michel in more detail.

Thomas was also in good spirits that afternoon. He was content and said that it had been a good year for him and his family. He talked a lot about the future prospects of his children. Over the years, he had invested a lot in education and further training for most of them, and he started to explain why he felt it had been a good year. Sylvie, his eldest daughter, then thirty-three years old, had finally completed a private course as a health assistant after several attempts to pass a similar course at the public nursing school. The private course had been expensive, but for Thomas it had been an important investment. The next step would be for Sylvie to pass a public exam in order to obtain a position within the public health care sector. Getting a job in the public sector in Burkina Faso would secure her a steady income, enabling her to care for herself, as she had not yet married. Although nurse aides receive a low salary, the job provides a regular income and comes with a pension, which provides some economic security during old age.

Myriel, the second oldest of the five daughters, was also at home, visiting her parents with her new, second pair of twins. She lived in a small town around forty kilometers from Keru. Thomas was very content that her future was secured: she was married and worked hard with her husband and in-laws to provide for their children. The third daughter, Caro, whose story opened this book, was also present. She had just given birth to her second child two days prior to this election day. Thomas expressed happiness about his new grandchildren, although he was worried about Caro's marriage. He also proudly told me that his two youngest daughters, Janine and Claudine, were doing very well in school. Janine completed her BEPC (*brevet d'études du premier cycle*) and was now studying for her BAC (baccalaureate) at a private school in another part of the province.[7]

Both Thomas and Beatrice had encouraged all their children to continue schooling, and a large share of their savings went to school fees and other related expenses. The two boys, Pascal and Michel, had not gone beyond primary school. During their childhood in the late 1990s, the local public school in Keru included only two classrooms, with about eighty children in each. At that time, the national school enrollment rate for children living in rural areas was only about 24 percent for boys and 14 percent for girls (DHS+ 2000; UNICEF 1998). The spoken language in school was French, a language that none of the children in Keru spoke at home. None of Thomas's boys, at that time, showed any particular interest in continuing their schooling. School enrollment has increased significantly since then. The existing school in Keru was expanded to include six classrooms and six teachers for a total of 350 enrolled children, and another public school was added to accommodate the growing number of children in the village.

Planning for the Future

Thomas felt that 2015 had been a good year for him and the family. Yet, he and Beatrice often discussed how best they could secure a good life for their family members. In 2019, when Thomas and I met at the local restaurant in Ouagadougou, it was clear that he had many thoughts about how to ensure a good life for all his children and a good old age for Beatrice and himself. Thomas expressed concern about how his sons would be able to take care of the farmland and ensure a good life for themselves and coming generations. He would soon have to hand over his obligations as head of the household to the next generation, but he worried about his children's prospects. Would they be able to seize opportunities to thrive and safeguard their future? Would the sons be able to take over and provide for Beatrice and himself once they were no longer were able to generate an income? At this moment in time, the family was in a critical phase of transition.

It worried Thomas a lot that Pascal was not yet married at the age of forty. The oldest son was supposed to take over as head of household, farm the family land, and take care of his parents, but Thomas wondered whether Pascal would be able to farm the land all by himself without a wife to help him, to cook, and to secure the next generation. Michel, the youngest son, had now spent almost five years in Libya. Thomas wanted him to come home despite the fact that Michel had not been able to earn enough to save or provide the family with remittances. Michel had also expressed a wish to return home. However, Thomas told me, he was caught in a "document trap," as he had neither a passport nor a *carte d'identité* with him in Libya. Without such proofs of identity, he would not be able to travel home legally. The whole family was worried about Michel, and although he regularly assured them that he was doing fine, they all feared for his safety and his future.

Sylvie, the oldest of the five daughters, was not married either. This also worried Thomas, as he would have liked to see all his daughters married off to husbands who would be able to provide for them. Sylvie had a child with a man who worked as a nurse in a nearby town. He was, however, already married and had not expressed any wish to divorce his wife or take a second wife. This bothered Thomas a lot. On the other hand, Sylvie had actually managed to pass the admission exam for the public sector health care position, and in 2019 she was posted at a health facility in the northern part of the country. While Thomas was quite happy about her job, he was concerned about the deteriorating security situation in the north. Her little daughter was staying with Thomas and Beatrice, and although they really enjoyed the company of their grandchildren, they were also worried about the child being separated from her mother, particularly since Sylvie did not know exactly how long she would be at her post.

Thomas now hoped that the two youngest daughters would succeed in becoming well-educated and would get jobs in the public sector. Janine had started studying history and archaeology at the University of Ouagadougou in 2018, and Thomas expressed his hopes for her future, saying, "I hope she will continue with studies, but how will we secure the means for her to continue? Thanks to God, I am still here. Our acquaintances said the university is far away and she needs a motorcycle. However, I asked an acquaintance of mine to accommodate her at a compound close to the university. So that's where she lives." Thomas continued, telling me that Janine had already signed up for one of the public sector *concours* (competitions) to become a public sector employee. "If she wins a competition, that's good," he explained. "It's a shortcut. These are BAC and BEPC level competitions. There is also the next who follows her, that is to say her little sister [Claudine]. She is also looking for the BAC. That's good." However, according to the newspapers, the chance of winning the competition was small, as an enormous number of people had signed up. In 2020, for example, 1,290,142 people signed up to participate in the exam to obtain one of 4,721 available posts![8]

Parents all over the world worry about the futures of their sons and daughters; however, being a subsistence farmer in rural Burkina Faso with little cash income poses many challenges for parents. Although most families in Keru now had a donkey and a cart to bring home agricultural products from the fields, most of the other work—sowing, weeding, and harvesting—was done manually. Few farmers had tractors, instead relying on oxen to plow the fields. Farmers could not produce enough surplus to purchase new equipment, and, because land was distributed according to customary law, it was almost impossible to acquire new land to farm. Most families therefore aimed to send one or more of their sons on *aventure*, primarily to other countries in West Africa to work on plantations or engage in other manual labor. However, as in the case of Thomas's sons, not all migrant workers succeed in getting jobs that allow them to send money home. Saving money in order to send the young men off or to support children's education required careful planning. For a father and head of household like Thomas, it was difficult to work out a strategy for improving the livelihood of the next generation in a context where harvests are notoriously unpredictable, where illness may be costly and debilitating, and where the children do not always want to follow their father's advice.

Encountering the State at the Polling Station

Casting a vote in national elections is one of the occasions where the state becomes visible to citizens of Burkina Faso. On election day in November 2015, Thomas and Beatrice had both cast their vote at the local school, which was transformed into a polling station under the supervision of the school's headmaster. Part of the excitement over this election was that Blaise Compaoré, who had been president for twenty-seven years, had fled the country after a popular uprising in response to his intention to change the constitution to permit him a third term as president. The new electoral code for the 2015 elections included procedures allowing independent candidates to stand for elections, providing financial support to party delegates in polling stations, and conducting a lottery in cases where candidates had the same number of votes and were the same age (Hagberg et al. 2018: 47–48). At this presidential election, a Bissa politician stood for the presidency among a number of other candidates.[9] According to Thomas, most people in this area supported the Bissa candidate and not Roch Marc Christian Kaboré, the presidential candidate of the MPP (Mouvement du Peuple pour le Progrès). The MPP, although it was a new party, was perceived by many as a continuation of Blaise Compaoré's old ruling party, the CDP (Congrès pour la Démocratie et le Progrès). When I passed by the polling station at the school just before it closed, the headmaster told me that they had registered 450 people, which was still less than 50 percent of the eligible voters. While the popular uprising against Blaise Compaoré had taken place primarily in Burkina Faso's urban centers, particularly in Ouagadougou and Bobo-Dioulasso, those in rural communities—including Thomas—had followed the process closely through radio and social media. I had listened to many discussions in Keru in which people expressed their discontent with Blaise Compaoré's initiative to change the constitution and their disappointment with his party.

As Veena Das has emphasized, most people encounter the state through documents such as birth and death certificates, identity cards, health booklets, criminal complaints, court papers, and ration cards. These documents bear the double sign of the state's distance and its penetration into everyday life. Through these documentary practices the state makes the population legible to itself, creating what has been referred to as a "legibility effect" (Auyero 2012; Das and Poole 2004: 15–16). An election day like this one was another point when citizens encountered the state. Becoming a voter in Burkina Faso was, however, not easy. It required quite a lot of paperwork. One needed to bring both a personal *carte d'identité* and an election card to the polling center. Citizens older than eighteen were eligible to obtain an election card, but getting it required showing one's birth certificate and identity card to the prefecture, where the election card would then be issued. Many people, particularly in the rural areas, did not have a birth certificate, and some did not have an identity card either, as these cards are primarily used when traveling. The eligibility of voters was, however, secured through these bureaucratic and rational procedures. Although it was complicated to be registered as a voter, people in Keru discussed the elections vigorously, and on election day many people expressed their satisfaction that a new president would be elected. Although most people were aware that their Bissa candidate had little chance of winning the election, they hoped it would bring some progress that would benefit more than a small urban political elite. About 60 percent of the registered voters cast their vote in 2015, compared to only 50 percent in 2020. The low participation rate in 2020 was partly caused by the closure of many polling stations in the northern part of the country due to security problems.[10]

Conclusion

Many changes have taken place in the village of Keru during the twenty-five years I have been engaged in this area. The size of the population has almost doubled.[11] The infrastructure has also improved: there is a new dispensary and an expanded school, and the village now has access to electricity. Also, the marketplace has grown, and more mosques and houses have been constructed, most using new types of material funded mainly by remittances from migrant work. However, the people of Keru continue to live precarious lives, despite the national economy growing around 5 to 6 percent annually during the last decade. The economic futures of individual family members continue to be fragile, but as the stories of Thomas and Beatrice and their seven children illustrate, situations of fragility and crisis also open up new possibilities: Michel had left for Libya, Sylvie got work in the northern part of the country, Janine studied at the university in Ouagadougou, and Thomas himself was constantly looking for opportunities to make some additional money by buying and selling livestock.

The most significant change, perhaps, is that the vast majority of people in the village now have a mobile phone or at least access to one. This was a big change, particularly for the many families whose relatives had migrated for work or were pursuing education in the urban areas. The mobile phone keeps people connected, which is especially important for those who stay behind, and that connection reminds migrants of family expectations concerning remittances. Such remittances continue to supplement subsistence agriculture, which remains the main economic activity in Keru.

As discussed in the introduction, the "absent-present" state, epitomized by almost-empty government facilities and low-quality services, coexisted with the "traditional" governance system. The Mossi kingdom maintained its influence in local politics, and the Bissa and Mossi village chiefs continued to play an important role in solving community disputes and organizing specific community activities. When I asked the local chief in Keru whether he thought there would still be a village chief in fifty years, he noted: "There will always be a need for someone to care for the village." Different systems sometimes coincided in the same person: for instance, Jean played an important role as a kind of "trickster," bridging traditional medical and ritual knowledge and practice with bureaucratic tasks, such as taking care of the water pumps and collecting taxes at the animal market.

Jean's generation had begun to pass away, and Thomas himself was aging, facing ongoing problems with hypertension. A few weeks after our conversation at the restaurant in Ouagadougou, Thomas was again admitted to the dispensary in Keru for observation. Persistent foot pain restricted him from tending his fields and made him anxious about what other diseases he might be suffering from. Thomas continued to worry about his sons: the eldest had a sore leg, which also hampered him from doing some of the hard agricultural work, and he was still unmarried. "Il est toujours enfant" (he is still a child), as Thomas said. He hoped that his youngest son would soon be able to return home from Libya and that his youngest daughters would make it through the educational system, eventually gaining employment in the public sector as *fonctionnaires* (public employees).

Notes

1. Italy has for many years been an important destination among Bissa migrants, although most Bissa migrate to other West African countries such as Côte d'Ivoire, Ghana, and Gabon.
2. The 2006 data were the most recent available from the secretariat at the municipality of Keru in 2020. A new national census was conducted in 2019, but the results were delayed due to the COVID-19 pandemic.
3. Index Mundi, "Burkina Faso Ethnic Groups," 18 September 2021. Retrieved 11 March 2023 from https://www.indexmundi.com/burkina_faso/ethnic_groups.html.
4. The language of the Mossi people, Mooré, belongs to a subdivision of the large group of Niger-Congo languages, called *gur* or *voltaïque*, while Bissa is categorized as a Mande language, which is another section of the Niger-Congo language family.
5. Also called Caro.
6. According to the *Encyclopedia Britannica*, a trickster is a protagonist who has magical powers and is characterized as a compendium of opposites. Encyclopedia Britannica, "Trickster Tale," 21 June 2017. Retrieved 15 October 2020 from https://www.britannica.com/art/trickster-tale.
7. Completion of the first six years of primary schooling in Burkina Faso results in the *certificat d'étude primaire* (CEP). Completing nine years of schooling results in the *brevet d'études du premier cycle* (BEPC). The baccalaureate is received after the eleventh year; university admission is possible after that time.
8. L'actualité du Burkina sur Internet, homepage. Retrieved 19 September 2020 from https://lefaso.net/.
9. Almost one hundred different parties, political formations, and independent groups were represented (Hagberg et al. 2018: 48).
10. Burkina Faso, Commission Electorale Nationale Independante (CENI), "Election presidentielle (1er tour), Resultat des voix obtenues par candidat." Retrieved June 2021 from https://www.ceni.bf/?q=content/r%C3%A9sultat-pr%C3%A9sidentielles-2015; Conseil Constitutionnel du Burkina Faso, "Elections." Retrieved 2 June 2021 from https://www.conseil-constitutionnel.gov.bf/elections.
11. As mentioned earlier, a new census was carried out in 2019. The final report came out in 2021 showing that the population had increased from 10.3 million in 1996 to 20.5 million in 2021. National Annual Statistics 2021. Retrieved 03 October 2023 from insd.bf/sites/default/files/2023-2/Annuaire_Statistique_National_2021.pdf. No census had been conducted between 2006 and 2019.

Chapter 2
Ambiguities of Child Care

> We could assume numerous forms. Many of us were birds. We knew no boundaries. There was much feasting, playing and sorrowing. We feasted much because of the beautiful terrors of eternity. We played much because we were free. And we sorrowed much because there were always those amongst us who had just returned from the world of the Living. They had returned inconsolable for all the love they had left behind, all the suffering they hadn't redeemed, all that they hadn't understood, and for all that they barely begun to learn before they were drawn back to the land of origins.
>
> —Ben Okri, *The Famished Road*

The Complicated Delivery

In the introduction, I recounted the story of the sudden death of Caro's baby boy. In this chapter, I explore how parents (and particularly mothers) of small children practice everyday health care. Exploring everyday childcare practices shows how demanding it is to do the care, how important it is to care for social relationships, and how fragile such relationships are. I argue that care work is not only hard and time-consuming but also involves careful cultivation of social relationships with relatives as well as with the spiritual world. This chapter also documents the ambiguities of childcare with a particular focus on how mothers juggle home treatments, consultations at public health facilities, and advice from local healers as they try to maintain the health of their small children, many of whom experience infectious diseases that leave them in a chronic state of sickness (Hänsch, Kroeker, and Oldenburg 2017; Sargent 1989).

Caro's delivery was complicated and took place under rather dramatic circumstances. I visited Caro at home in her in-law's compound just four days after the delivery in 2015, but it was only a year later, when she told me the full story of the sudden death of her child, that I understood why the delivery ended up being so difficult and strenuous. Caro's story illustrates the intricacies of neonatal and maternal health care in rural Burkina Faso. This is not only due to a weak and poorly equipped health care system but also because health care services, although available, are not always easy to access. The public services are, in a sense, both present and absent for young women such as Caro. Her position in the household of her in-laws was precarious, and she did not have any of her own income to pay for treatment or care at the hospital, had she wanted it. The dispensary was not physically distant, but she did not see it as accessible for her. The story of the sudden death of Caro's child also demonstrates that complex and delicate family relations may affect healthcare-seeking practices and highlights serious allegations about witchcraft that may occur among in-law families.

Caro's voice was weak and trembling when she talked about the childbirth at our conversation a few days after the delivery, and she spoke in short sentences:

> I delivered Thursday afternoon at around 3 p.m. When I woke up in the morning, the pains in my stomach started. I did not deliver at the hospital. I delivered at home. It was only after the delivery that somebody called my husband, and he came and took me to the hospital [dispensary]. When we arrived, the nurse put her gloves on and removed the remaining blood in my stomach. After that, she gave me an injection and she gave me a bed, where we stayed for two days. Then, Saturday evening we were sent home.

Caro looked pale and tired. The mother-in-law was also present during this conversation. After Caro's brief description of the delivery, the mother-in-law started telling her part of the story. She told us that she and Caro had been quarreling that morning. Caro had therefore locked herself up in her little room and closed the venetian blinds of the single small window. Caro was inside the room in almost total darkness, giving birth to her son without any assistance. The mother-in-law had returned from the field, prepared her lunch, and eaten, only then realizing that Caro was delivering her baby inside the locked room. She tried to persuade Caro to open the door. After the delivery, Caro eventually unlocked the door because she was worried that the newborn boy was not crying as he was supposed to. The mother-in-law entered the room and discovered that the child was still covered by the amniotic sac. She managed to remove the amniotic sac and cut the cord, which was around the child's neck and one of his legs. After the mother-in-law had liberated the baby from the amniotic sac, he started to breathe normally. The mother-in-law went ahead to the dispensary with the baby. The nurse there asked the mother-in-law where the child's mother was and told her to immediately bring Caro to the dispensary, as otherwise she risked dying. While the mother-in-law organized transport to the dispensary, Caro washed and prepared herself. They managed to get in touch with Caro's husband, who took her to the dispensary on the back of his motorcycle. Caro and the baby were admitted to the dispensary for two days. Both Caro and her mother-in-law agreed about the story up to this point.

Caro continued the story and explained that she had used some herbal medicine to reduce the pain while she was in labor (not in order to speed up the birth, as documented in other studies from this area, such as Østergaard [2015]). She had not taken any other medicine besides this. At the dispensary, she received one injection and was given a prescription for paracetamol and amoxicillin. After the conversation, which took place outside of Caro's small house, in the courtyard, I was invited to step inside the house to see the newborn. He was lying on a thick layer of *pagne* (cloth) on the floor of the house, looking at us and waving his arms and legs in uncontrolled movements as newborns often do.

I was puzzled about the events surrounding the child's birth, and many questions came to mind as we drove back to Keru. Why had Caro locked herself up in a small, dark room? Why did she give birth to a child without assistance from anybody? The mother-in-law might be a good woman, but, according to Thomas, she had the habit of quarreling when drunk. What had they been arguing about that morning? Why did Caro not prepare herself to go to the dispensary for the delivery? I could not figure it out. Perhaps she was upset about the quarrel with her mother-in-law, perhaps she had prior bad experiences with the dispensary, or perhaps she was afraid that the dispensary would demand payment for services. She did not clearly explain why she made the choices she had, but it was clear that both she and her baby had been at great risk during this fragile delivery. During my conversation with Caro about ten months after the death of the child, she told us that during his two and a half months of life, the boy had not been ill with any unusual illness and was not ill before his sudden death. However, Caro told us that he used to cry a lot, especially at night. He could cry for an hour, then after being breastfed, he would sleep, but later he would wake up again and cry. He had gained weight and had looked fine, Caro explained.

The story of the death of Caro's baby was sad and confusing. During our conversations, Caro made it clear that it had never been a happy marriage and that she felt lonely. Her husband was seldom at home, and the mother-in-law, despite being a Christian,[1] supported her son's opinion about the children's religious upbringing. This conflict in their marriage went deep and involved more than just the couple. The two families obstinately accused each other of being responsible for the death of the child.

> *Caro*: The child died because my mother-in-law performed a lot of sacrifices. Every time, she hailed ancestors to take the life of the child. When we were together, she talked only about that. She made it a topic of discussion. My own mother, she also refused, saying that I should not stop going to the church. These are the explanations of the death of the child. The child did not fall ill before dying.

Caro found herself in an existential dilemma. She wanted to continue to belong to the Catholic Church, and she also wanted her children to belong to the church. Her parents and siblings were active members of the local church: Thomas had served as a catechist for many years, and the family had attended Sunday services and special events in the church throughout Caro's childhood. She could not leave her religion, she explained. On the other hand, she was afraid of her mother-in-law and afraid of the power she had.

> *Helle*: What type of sacrifice did your mother-in-law do?
>
> *Caro*: She did the sacrifices to the ancestors of her home village. She says, those ancestors, her parents.
>
> *Helle*: How did she do the sacrifices?
>
> *Caro*: She did the incantations. She went to eat the fetishes. While eating the fetishes, she spoke to the ancestors, and they listened to her (*Elle est*

> *allée bouffer des fétiches. En bouffant les fétiches, quand elle parle aux ancêtres, ils entendent*).[2] If, for example, she says that you will die today, her wishes will be executed. My mother-in-law says that if a person offends her and she wants that person to die, it is enough for her to consume the fetish and the person who has insulted her will die immediately. If my mother-in-law says that you will die tomorrow, you will effectively die tomorrow. Otherwise, she will sacrifice a chicken to the ancestors asking them to comply with a vow. The person who has offended her can avoid the death only on the condition that the person offers apologies to my mother-in-law. Even before the delivery of my child, my mother-in-law said that I would have a miscarriage. If not, the child would die at birth. That is the reason why I asked my mother-in-law to forgive me. She let me know that she had accepted the apologies, and she did not do anything at that time. I know that if she goes to her home [village] she will ask the ancestors to kill the child.

Although official policy strongly recommends that pregnant women go to a public health facility for delivery, Caro had delivered her son at home. A public dispensary was located only a few kilometers from Caro's home, but she had not thought of it as accessible to her. When the child did not react as expected after birth, the mother-in-law took the child to the dispensary herself. Caro was brought to the dispensary only after the nurse insisted that she be brought to the dispensary, as her health could be in danger after the difficult delivery.

It was only after the conversation with Caro ten months after the death of her son that I understood the extent of Caro's misery and the dilemmas she faced. Even before the delivery of the child, Caro had feared that her mother-in-law would harm the baby. According to Caro, the mother-in-law had several times told her that the child would die during pregnancy, through miscarriage, or during the delivery. This may have been why Caro had locked herself up and decided to deliver the baby all alone in a dark room. When Caro told me the story of the sudden death of her child, she was clearly scared and bewildered. Facing a complex dilemma, she expressed qualms about what to do. She was afraid of living in the same household with her husband and mother-in-law, and she was afraid that her now five-year-old daughter also was in danger of being bewitched by her husband's family.

According to Caro herself, she was trapped in a religious conflict between her husband's wish that she should convert to Islam, his insistence that their children should follow his faith, and her own strong attachment to the Catholic Church. The couple was also quarreling about each other's contributions to the household. Due to a severe eye infection during her teenage years, for which she still needed treatment, Caro had difficulty working in the field, as the dust and strong sun were harmful to her eyes. The husband wanted her to work more in the field, which she was unable to do, and she claimed that he never did any labor himself and that he mainly lived off one of his brothers, who worked as a nurse in the nearby town. Caro had also found herself in a dilemma in relation to her own family of origin, as her father had insisted that she marry her husband, despite their huge age difference. In one of our conversations, Caro said that it had been "a forced marriage," while Thomas claimed that Caro herself had accepted the marriage proposal from her husband. Thomas was, according to Caro, afraid that she would end up like her elder sister, having a child but no husband. Getting by as a divorced, single mother is not easy in a rural community. It is considered shameful, and it would therefore be difficult to find a new husband. Furthermore, moving back to her parents' household would be a defeat for the whole family. Such a situation would challenge Thomas's role as a father able to establish good relations with his children's in-laws. Economically, it was not easy for Thomas either, as he was already struggling to make ends meet, as only one of his adult daughters was married and integrated into an in-law family. For Caro, caring for her children and bringing them up in a moral universe that she believed in was much harder than she had expected. She had lost one child, and she was seriously afraid that her five-year-old daughter was also in danger.

I do not have the full story from the husband's or the mother-in-law's perspective, but it is beyond doubt that the sudden death of the child had shattered Thomas and his family. They were a family of devoted Christians, and during my many interviews with traditional healers (including witchcraft specialists), Thomas always kept himself in the background. Jean, Thomas's relative, introduced me to the various specialists practicing traditional medicine in Keru and the surrounding villages. Thomas clearly faced a dilemma in reconciling traditional animistic perceptions and practices and his Christian belief. In this case of the sudden death of Caro's child, however, he claimed that it had to be a case of witchcraft.

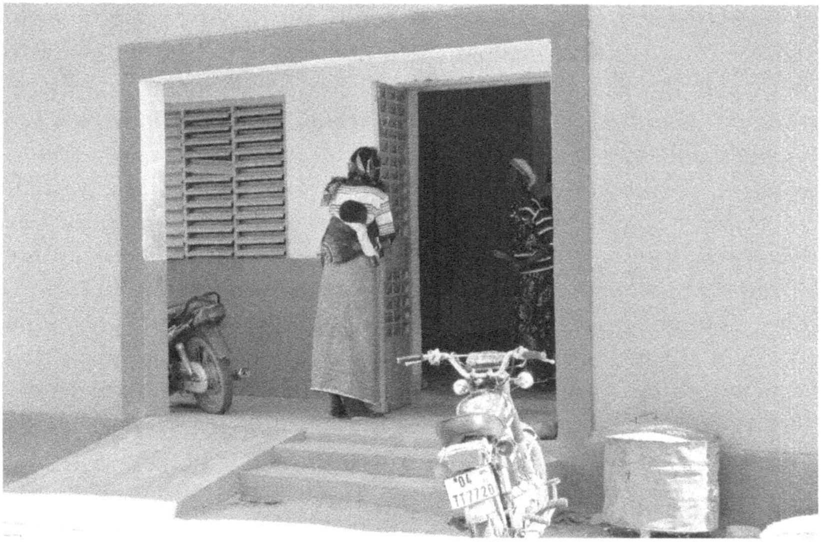

Figure 2.1. Mother and baby in front of a dispensary, Burkina Faso (© Helle Samuelsen 2023)

Care Ethics in Childcare

Babies and small children depend on comprehensive care during their first years of life to secure food and shelter and to ensure their development and socialization (Barnes 2012; Gottlieb 2004; Scheper-Hughes 2014). Basic survival depends on care, and care is fundamentally a relational activity. Analyzing childcare, as I do in this chapter, requires exploring the social relationships small children are part of. Such an examination shows how fragile the lives of small children are in rural Burkina Faso. The sudden death of Caro's child illustrated this in excruciating ways, as the death elicited a mix of matrimonial and religious conflict between the two families. Recriminations concerning the cause of the child's death were expressed by both families. Caro and the rest of her family accused the mother-in-law of causing the child's death through witchcraft. The mother-in-law and her family, in turn, accused Caro of causing the death of the child herself.

In what follows, I examine the mundane, everyday practices of care that mothers undertake in Keru. This includes both the mothers' efforts to keep diseases away from their small children as well as their caring practices when children fall ill. As Iain Wilkinson and Arthur Kleinman explain, "Through care we are equipped to participate in social life, and in being cared for we are affirmed with recognition and value. In acts of care real things are at stake, including life itself" (2016: 161). I draw here on the notion of care ethics, which takes its point of departure in the perception that the world is comprised of human relations rather than of people standing alone (Robinson 1997: 120). Knud Ejler Løgstrup notes that human life is "not first solitary, and then, as if by accident, lived together with other human beings" (Løgstrup 1991: 144). Rather, a person's life always is entangled with the lives of others. Løgstrup claims that "who we are and how we live is, to an unfathomable extent, dependent upon our involvement with others" (Fink 2007: 12; Løgstrup 1997). In Løgstrup's thinking, relationality and dependency are extensive and deep. The person-to-person relationship is one of the most important aspects of human life. For Løgstrup, the "ethical" refers to the demand to act unselfishly for the best interests of each of the other people who trust in us (Fink 2007: 15; Løgstrup 1997). It is a prima facie demand—implicit, unarticulated, and silent (Fink 2007: 16). Paul Ricoeur's ethics makes a similar point, emphasizing that care is relational (Kearney 1996; Van Nistelrooij, Schaafsma, and Tronto 2014). In his terminology, *care* includes both the practices of treating a sick person well and recognizing the individual patient's singular worth. Ricoeur encourages a focus on practice and highlights the importance of understanding the relationship between action and agent in the production of ethical practice. He claims that ethics often overemphasizes "the what" and "the why" and insufficiently understands "the who" undertaking the action in question (Carney 2015; Kingori 2013; Ricoeur 1994: 58–60; Van Nistelrooij et al. 2014). Ricoeur's conceptualization calls attention to the immense workload of care that mothers in rural Burkina Faso (and beyond) carry out as part of everyday life and brings to the fore their enormous, often tacit responsibilities, not least during periods where their husbands are absent due to migration.

The importance of care as a relational practice is obvious when, as in this case, we study infants and children, who depend on years of deep care. This chapter also demonstrates the importance of focusing on the "who"—here mothers are the principal caregivers. The case of Caro's baby elucidates how broken relations between caregivers may be fatal for small children. Caring is also fundamental in other phases of life during the life course, not least in times of illness (Barnes 2012b: 13). Care ethics emphasizes the relations between the caregiver and the recipient of care, focusing on the practical and the affective more than on the normative. Care work, as I use it here, is grounded in everyday practice, the *doing* of care (Mol 2008), and often includes brute materiality, as Wilkinson and Kleinman stress: "heavy lifting, physical support, and hard work. It exacts a heavy bodily and emotional toll on those doing it. It is a painstaking activity that requires considerable commitments of physical energies and a readiness to involve oneself in troubled and conflicted emotional situations" (2016: 162). The care that children receive when ill shows how care ethics is highly gendered in rural Burkina Faso. Women are primarily responsible for care work carried out in the household. Men become involved primarily when there is a need for transport of sick family members to public health care facilities, as we saw in the case of Caro's delivery, and when dealing with payment for health services. In chapters 6 and 7, I discuss the relationship between citizens and the state in more detail, asking questions about the responsibility of the state to take care of its citizens. Here, I restrict my focus to the responsibilities within the close family, particularly the relationship between the young child and the primary caregiver, who in the case of infants and children under five is generally the child's mother.

In addition to the examination of care as practice, I also want to emphasize the importance of understanding the structural position of women and the often fragile positions they have within the family. Mothers exercise a lot of agency and make many day-to-day decisions concerning household tasks, including caring for sick or vulnerable family members, but they are structurally dependent on their husbands or other male members of the household. Care relations are intrinsically fragile in this part of the world, particularly when caregivers themselves have restricted access to education, employment, health services, and other social goods. However, as mentioned above, situations of fragility and uncertainty also open up the possibility for new actions in the search for a good life.

For Ricoeur, acting and suffering are interconnected, but, as he says, "we must go further and take into account more deeply concealed forms of suffering: the incapacity to tell a story, the refusal to recount, the insistence of the untellable" (Ricoeur 1994: 320; Savage 2013). Ricoeur might not have thought of rural African mothers when writing this, but it applies to them as well. Because of their often inferior position in the family, much of their care work remains invisible and unrecognized. Maimouna, one of the more outspoken women who had remained in the village while her husband worked for years in Equatorial Guinea, expressed her discontent with her husband's apparent ignorance about the hard work she did. When asked whether she had any problems during her husband's absence, she replied: "It is not small problems, I have. When I say that there are difficulties, it is because there are certain things that the husband should support. He should care for his wife, he should take care of the medical treatment of his wife, when ill. Since he went to Guinea, I sometimes call him, but he does not answer. Sometimes, he complains saying that you don't behave well." Maimouna continued: "I make a living from my small business and farming. Besides the business and the farming, there is nothing else. When I have problems, my brothers will come and help me. When I was ill, it was my own brothers and my mother who treated me at the district hospital until I recovered. Then I went back to the village and took care of the children." In these quotes, Maimouna expressed a feeling of being let down by her husband, as well as frustration about his inability to recognize her needs and her daily care work.

The Liminality of Young Children

The child mortality rate in Burkina Faso was estimated to be 85 of every thousand live births in 2019.[3] In other words, almost one child out of eleven died before his or her fifth birthday. In 1994, the rate was 198 for every thousand live births—that is, almost a fifth of all children died before the age of five. Over the twenty-five years from 1994 to 2019, the child mortality rate declined by more than half. This is in many ways an impressing decrease, although the country did not reach the Millennium Development Goal of 67 per thousand live births by 2015. Too many children continue to suffer from illness and die. Among fifty women I interviewed in 2010, twenty-one reported that they had experienced at least one child death, and ten had experienced more than one child death. Malaria, upper respiratory infections such as pneumonia, and diarrheal diseases are among the most common illnesses (Institut National de la Statistique et de la Démographie 2021), and about 72 percent of children under five suffer from anemia. Families in Burkina Faso are clearly confronted with many serious health care challenges, and recurrent child illnesses form part of everyday life.

In his analysis of the socialization of Mossi children, Amadé Badini distinguishes between different phases of childhood and their associated childcare practices (Badini 1994). The first phase starts at conception and ends at birth. Here, as in most other societies, there are rules about how pregnant woman should ensure a good delivery and a healthy child: what they should and should not do, what they should and should not eat. During my fieldwork, I heard about many dangers, rules, and taboos related to pregnant women. Quite a few of them relate to perceived dangers of the bush (*la brousse*), the area outside the village. One traditional healer explained that if a *margouillat* (lizard) touches the feet of a pregnant woman, the child would get a disease called *margouillat*, losing weight and becoming frail. Thomas's relative Jean,[4] who was very knowledgeable about the flora and fauna of the region, explained that pregnant women should be careful not to cross the track of a python, as the mother or the unborn child would risk catching a disease called *waofo* (python snake). It might take up to a year before the disease would emerge, with snake-like spots on the skin and partial paralysis. If a woman is less than eight months pregnant, the mother would miscarry or the child would be stillborn; if she is more than eight months pregnant, the child will be born but will eventually develop the disease, which Jean claimed to be relatively common in this area. He stressed that only the python causes this disease; other snakes make sinuous tracks in the sand, while pythons make straight tracks. If a person notices such tracks in the sand, he or she should immediately find a stick and erase the snake track. Sylvie Fainzang found similar explanations among the Bissa around Garango. She described how it is thought that the sight of a python might cause the disease called *wafo*, which causes spots on the skin. According to Fainzang, it is not viewing the snake that transmits the disease; the python is an animated spirit, and such a disease would never be transmitted by accident. The python makes itself visible when something wrong has happened. Thus, the disease is a kind of sanction due to the person's inappropriate act (Fainzang 1986: 71). In addition to concerns about snake tracks, the Bissa, as is the case in many other cultures, also have many food restrictions. For example, pregnant women should avoid eating sweet mangoes or other sweet fruits. In addition, they should not eat too much fresh meat, and both pregnant and lactating women should avoid pork, chicken, and goat meat.

According to the local cosmology, small children are in a liminal state between the human world into which they are born and the spiritual world from which they originate. After birth, the newborn should be kept indoors for the first seven days as a protective measure. Furthermore, babies should never be left alone: they are either carried on the back of the mother (or the back of a sister) or taken care of by other family members. During my first few months of fieldwork in Keru in 1996, I spent a lot of time with the family of Thomas and Beatrice. Their youngest child, Michel, was fourteen months old at the time. Following the family on an almost daily basis, I noticed that illness among small children was part of everyday life. On 23 September, I made the following notes in my notebook:

> Beatrice sits outside under the *hangar* [shelter] with her little son, Michel. He is ill with fever and has vomited twice within the last couple of hours. It is *le palu* (malaria), they say. According to Beatrice, it is the fifth time he suffers from *palu* within his short lifetime—and the other children have also each suffered from *palu* once or twice this year. They have given him some Aspirin in order to reduce the fever. No wonder that some of the children of the village look small and frail. Thomas says that his illness came after he played in the water last Thursday after the heavy rains.

If Michel suffered from *palu* five times in fourteen months and each of the other four children had also been ill a couple of times, that means the children had at least thirteen episodes of illness in a years' time, more than one new case of sickness every month. A week later, on 1 October, I noted that Michel remained sick:

> Michel feels warm when touching his head, and he is very quiet. They (Beatrice and Thomas) explain that since Beatrice has diarrhea (due to changes in the diet), her breastmilk is passing the illness to Michel. Later during the day, she gives him some Paracetamol diluted in water, which he, however, is not keen on swallowing—and which he expeditiously vomits again.

On 3 October, Michel is still ill:

> He has fever and they say that he is vomiting and has diarrhea, however, he eats a little and he is breastfeeding. Beatrice thinks it is *palu*, malaria. It is the water of the rainy season, she explains, there are small streams of water on the ground after the heavy rains, and when he plays in the water, he happens to swallow some of the water. It is the water that causes his illness *hihel* (literally meaning "water" in Bissa). They have given him Aspirin and some yellow tablets/pills imported from Ghana (bought at the local market in Keru). Thomas buys, later the same day, Nivaquine (malaria medicines) to give to Michel.

On 8 October, I made a note in my notebook that Michel is well again. The illness lasted a couple of weeks. During this episode, the family had tried various medicines, but they did not consult the health care system. The nearest dispensary at that time was located in Tenga, about three kilometers from Keru. Cases of fever among Thomas and Beatrice's children, as with most other children in Keru, are part of everyday life. The most common symptoms among small children are fever, diarrhea, and cough. The parents are worried and pay a lot of attention to a sick child but going to a public health facility is not necessarily their first move.

Paying attention to the well-being of small children is important, not only because they depend on everyday caregiving from mothers and other relatives, but also because they are in a liminal state between the world of the spirits and the human world, as the quote at the beginning of this chapter from Ben Okri's novel, *The Famished Road*, illustrates. In Mooré, *Saana* is a term used to describe children in the transitional period from birth to about three years, when breastfeeding is terminated. *Saana* means "the stranger" and conveys small children's ambivalent position: the newborn arrives in the world of the living as unknown and not a priori recognized. The teeth are the first hard substances to emerge, and only at this point does the child's relationship with the spiritual world diminish. Language development is another important sign of the small child's disengagement from the spiritual world (Bonnet 1988: 71). Thomas was worried about Michel's language development and believed that he was not developing language skills as he was supposed to. Thomas mentioned this to me quite a few times when Michel, at the age of two, communicated primarily with one-syllable words and other sounds. During one of my later visits to Burkina Faso, Thomas told me, with relief in his voice, that Michel had now developed his language skills appropriately.[5]

A mother's attention and care are extremely important during the fragile transitional period between birth and three to four years of age, as scholars in various parts of West Africa have observed. Among the Papel of Guinea-Bissau, Jónína Einarsdóttir reported that children were either born as a reincarnated person (*pekadar*), a human being with the soul of a person who had already died, or as a non-human being, a spirit (*iran*). The few non-human children whom Einarsdóttir encountered during her fieldwork were visibly different from normal children—a couple of them had physical impairments, others were severely paralyzed, and one was seriously malnourished. Among the Papel, a woman risked giving birth to a non-human child if she bathed naked at a spring with running water. The spirit might be attracted to the woman and enter her womb, thereby hindering a human soul from entering it (Einarsdóttir [2000] 2004). Alma Gottlieb emphasized that among the Beng in Côte d'Ivoire, infants were believed to understand all languages spoken by humans. As they slowly disassociated themselves from *wrugbe*, the spiritual world, they lost their ability to understand all languages and came to specialize in their own "native" language (Gottlieb 2004: 98). Katherine M. Dettwyler's study of childcare in Magnambougou, Mali, also emphasized the relationship between small children and spirits. Here, pregnant women had to be cautious when walking in the bush at night, as evil spirits might "take over" the child. If a bad spirit succeeded, the child could be born dead or deformed—or it might never grow up. If a child never grew or stopped growing, never reaching out for things or walking or talking, it was not a real child but an evil spirit that eventually would transform itself into a snake and slither away (Dettwyler 1993: 85–86). Among the Mossi, all newborns were perceived as "ontological cuttings" of a forefather who had returned among the living through the *kinkirga*, the twin spirit (Badini 1994: 47). Traditionally, conception was perceived as the work of the spirits when a *kinkirga* entered the woman during intercourse.

In the village of Keru, it is the responsibility of the parents, particularly mothers, to anticipate and protect a young child against danger. Mothers have to pay special attention to their children's well-being in order to ensure that they remain in the human world and refrain from going back to the world of the spirits. The liminal period of early childhood is characterized by a number of rituals as well as everyday dos and don'ts that mothers should follow (V. Turner 1967; Van Gennep 2013). For example, mothers carry their small children on their backs when they work in the fields, when they go to the market, and when they cook at home. By doing so, mothers are able to protect their children from many threats, including those in the bush area outside the village.

A traditional healer told me that mothers with small babies should be careful in the bush. If they encountered a hare, the child risked falling sick with very high fever. The sickness would be transmitted to the child through the eyes. It would be an insult to the child if this taboo were trespassed, the healer said. By using the word "insult," she emphasized that small children needed to be cared for and respected. Control of bodily thresholds was also important in daily preventive and therapeutic practices, such as purging small children regularly with herbal decoctions. The fontanel was also seen as an orifice: wind or cold air could enter the body through the fontanel and cause a sickness called *zugu* (Chandler et al. 2015).[6] One woman explained that if the child's head were not well protected early in the morning, the wind would enter the child. As a result, the respiration of the fontanel would stop and the child would become seriously ill. Most small children were protected from this illness by wearing knitted caps (Samuelsen 1999: 73–80).

There were also a number of guidelines regarding the diet of the breastfeeding mother, as is common in many other cultures. A traditional healer explained that he treated a disease called *gôonré*, a disease of the stomach in which the feces became yellowish but changed to greenish when exposed to the air. This disease was related to the mother's diet during pregnancy; if she consumed too much fatty and succulent food and then failed to purge the child using an enema of water and bitter herbs at birth, the child would suffer from this disease. A traditional birth attendant, who was also an expert in treating a number of diseases and managed a restaurant in the Keru market, told me about another guideline: if a woman had lost her previous child, she needed to wash herself with a specific concoction of leaves from the bush in order to ritually free herself from the impurity of the dead child. If this was not done, the new child would risk falling ill from *kaam*, an illness in which the child becomes pale (white), loses weight, and has a dry mouth. Knowledge about how to give proper care to small children and how to avoid the many threats was passed from mother to daughter and from mother-in-law to daughter-in-law. In addition, when their own expertise was insufficient to address illness, many mothers consulted local specialists with specific knowledge and skills related to childcare. These specialists were often elders gifted with knowledge about dangers caused by troubled relationships with the spiritual world or problematic social relationships that could cause illness (Samuelsen 1999).

Enemas in Everyday Health Care

During my first months of fieldwork in 1996, I noticed that small bulb syringes, similar to those typically used for cleaning ears or aspirating nasal passages, were left casually on the low walls or on the ground in many households. After some time, I realized that small children were given enemas on a regular basis and that the small pumps were used for this purpose. Infants were given enemas daily, and small children up to the age of two to three years were also given them regularly. The consistent use of enemas in childcare was accompanied by a number of other caring practices that revealed a strong concern for children's health and the many risks that threaten it. Michel was also given enemas a few times every week during his first years. According to many of the mothers and local herbalists I spoke with, the enemas were used for cleansing and preventing diseases. Often, the enemas only included lukewarm water, but sometimes water was mixed with herbs such as *siiga*, *taanga* (*karité*), *gaga*, and *kuelenga*. Sometimes enemas were also used to "inject" the child's medicines. The small pumps were convenient for these purposes, as previously mothers used their mouths to blow water into the child. The enemas also helped mothers to control the defecation of their small children, which is practical in this part of the world, where disposable diapers are still not available. Instead of diapers, mothers usually carry an extra piece of *pagne*, which is used to catch urine when the child is carried around and when the child is sitting in someone's lap. It is perceived to be embarrassing if the child urinates or defecates on "strangers." I have many times been sitting with a baby on my lap while chatting with village women, who always made sure that a piece of *pagne* was placed under the baby (see also Gottlieb 2004: 132–33). Giving an enema is a particular expression of care for newborns and small children. It involves quite a lot of effort to collect the herbs, boil and cool the decoction, and provide the enemas.

Koom: A Disease of the Youngest Child

Fever, as mentioned above, was the most common symptom of illness among small children in Keru. *Koom* (Bissa: *Hihel*), a Mooré term that literally means water, is one of several illnesses characterized by fever. The primary symptom was fever, but the hands, feet, and buttocks of those suffering from *koom* also got cold. Locally, it was a common diagnosis used by mothers, often described as a type of *palu* (or malaria, from French: *paludisme*). Only the youngest sibling could get this disease, as many mothers of small children told me. Most could not explain why this disease only attacked the youngest in a family, but they assured me that it was a fact. The disease was, in principle, not related to a specific age group; even adults could get the disease if they were the youngest sibling. Beatrice explained it this way: "During the rainy season, the children suffer from *palu* and *koom*. It may happen that *koom* attacks adults if they are the Benjamins of their mother[7]. For example, you, you are the youngest of your mother's children, the *koom* malaria could strike you, here in Africa. The *koom* strikes the last, or the last born of a mother, even if the last born is adult, even old, the *koom* only attacks the last born." Beatrice continued: "You know, it's a kind of *palu*; it can also bring diarrhea and vomiting. . . . To protect a child from *koom*, all women take a small amount of mud and place it on the head of the child when passing a stream in order to prevent the *koom*." I only heard about *koom* during the rainy seasons, and I only heard about *koom* in cases of small children who caught the disease when playing in the puddles of rainwater. Mamouna, a female traditional healer, explained *koom* in the following way:

> It is the spirits of the small children who died recently, who return and reside in the water streams during the rainy season. It is they who try to drown the living children. This is what carries along the *koom* disease during the rainy season. They enjoy it most when the children have a lot of hair. They drop the child into the water puddles and hold it up by its feet. When the child has a lot of hair, the water will drip for a long time.

> This is what they enjoy most; they say that their claypot/bowl is full and will take long before it dries out. (Interview, 1997)

As mentioned above, Michel suffered from *koom* during my first period of fieldwork in the village, and Beatrice referred to his playing in puddles as an explanation of his illness, saying, "Do you remember, one time Michel played on the ground, when you were about to leave, and two days later, he got the *koom*. He played in the flow of water; it was after that he caught this illness." That only the youngest in a family could catch this disease conveys their liminality, emphasizing that the last born needed particular attention and protection.

Care Labor

Adissa, a young mother in her early twenties, lived with her in-laws in Keru, though her husband was based in Côte d'Ivoire. Her three children often fell ill; the two eldest children, five years and three years old, respectively, often suffered from *sobgo* (literally "wind"; often translated as *palu*/malaria), which according to Adissa was caused by food as well as wind. When they fell ill, she usually bought some paracetamol at the local market to give them. She also collected a number of bush plants, which she first boiled and then used for bathing the children, treating them for at least three days in a row. The youngest child, who was six months old, suffered from *tiisi* face spots and an eye infection. During this illness, Adissa had both consulted a local herbal specialist and visited the dispensary. In addition, the youngest child had over a period of ten days suffered from *yingwingre* (warm body), which according to Adissa was caused by the sun. She had consulted the dispensary, and the child had eventually recovered from this case of illness. Taking care of three small children who often fell ill involved not only a lot of speculation and reflection about how best to protect them and treat them, but also a lot of physical activity, searching for specific plants to use in the herbal treatments, preparing the decoctions, visiting the market to buy medicines, seeking advice from herbal specialists, and consulting the dispensary. All this in addition to the "soft work" of comforting the children when they were ill. As I observed practices of caregiving in Keru and neighboring villages over a period of more than twenty years, I could see mothers' constant attentiveness, their continuous agency, and their flexible responses to symptoms affecting their small children. Caring for the young is hard work. While public health care services were not far away in geographical terms, they were, for various reasons, not always accessible, and not always considered relevant to consult.

I have mainly focused on the relationship between mothers and their small children; however, this does not imply that fathers have no important roles. Often, decisions about the treatment of ill children are made jointly by the parents, and consulting public health care facilities, where payment is expected, requires consent and often money from the father or, in the absence of the father, other male members of the household. However, most fathers have little to do with ordinary domestic life (Laugier 2015), the minute-by-minute routine activities of childcare such as feeding, bathing, carrying, and cleaning. As most mothers work hard all day, cooking, washing, and tending the fields, other family members might also be involved in the everyday care work of children. When children reach four or five years of age, they sometimes stay for up to several weeks with other family members, particularly if the mother has conceived again. For example, one of the twin children of Myriel (one of Thomas and Beatrice's daughters), a girl about four years old, stayed with her

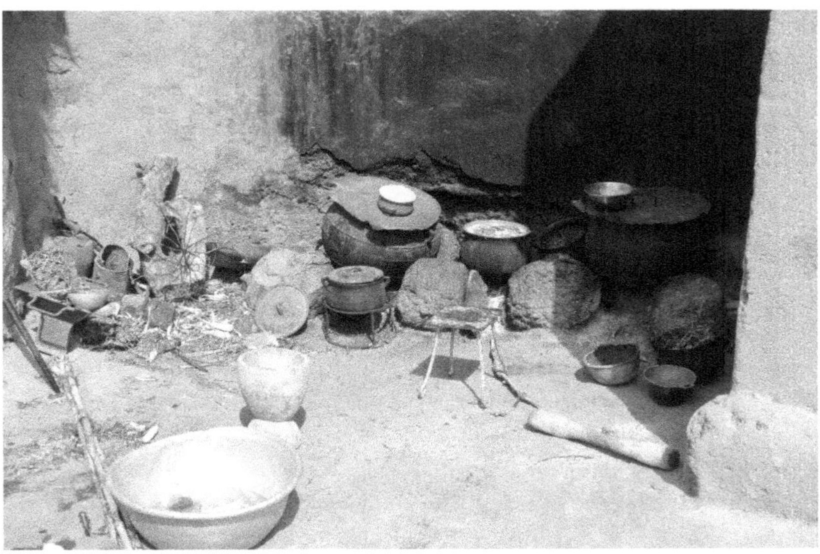

Figure 2.2. Kitchen in a rural household, Burkina Faso (© Helle Samuelsen 2023)

grandparents after Myriel gave birth to another set of twins. The small girl had bonded closely with Thomas, although he told me that by the end of the three-week visit, she asked him every day when she would go back to live with her mother.

As Wilkinson and Kleinman point out, when "questioning what care involves people doing, the conditions under which care is practiced, who does the care work, and how well particular individuals and groups are cared for, we are set to examine the most elemental conditions of human sociality" (Wilkinson and Kleinman 2016: 161). This type of work corresponds well to Hannah Arendt's notion of *labor*, which she defines as "the activity which corresponds to the biological process of the human body, whose spontaneous growth, metabolism, and eventual decay are bound to the vital necessities produced and fed into the life process by labor. The human condition of labor is life itself" (2013: 7). For Arendt, labor is "the daily fight in which the human body is engaged to keep the world clean and prevent its decay. . . . [T]he endurance it needs to repair every day anew the waste of yesterday is not courage, and what makes the effort painful is not danger but its relentless repetition" (2013: 101). The care work, or the physical and emotional *labor* mothers do every day, demands agency as well as endurance. It is characterized both by repetition, as Arendt emphasizes, but also, as we have seen above, by trial and error and improvisation (Livingston 2012).

Following children's illnesses over time illustrates the immense workload caregivers invest in improving the health of their children. Kabiro, a young child less than four years old, had suffered from fever, diarrhea, and nausea since the start of the rainy season a few months earlier. At our first interview, Setou, his grandmother, told me that they started treatment by collecting small branches from five different trees.[8] The branches were soaked in water for five days, and the child was bathed and washed with this water. They had also consulted the pensioned nurse, Dr. Sorgho, at his home clinic in the village, where the child was given a total of six injections (two injections a day for three days) and some medicines, which they diluted in warm water and used to purge the child. They also consulted the dispensary in Tenga, where the child was admitted for five days and received another set of injections and medicines. The grandmother remarked at the first interview that "since it is not a baby, we have not consulted the old healers." She was convinced that the child had fallen ill because he did not want a new sibling, as his illness started when his mother got pregnant again.

When we visited one week later, the grandmother told us that Kabiro was feeling better, but that he was still vomiting and feverish. They had not, however, given him any new herbal or pharmaceutical medicines. In the third week, the grandmother informed us that Kabiro was not vomiting anymore but continued to have diarrhea. They had searched for a specific bark (*Sambnoré* in Mooré), which they had boiled and used to purge him. They had not consulted anybody, as "money is short." In the fourth week, the mother said that the disease had relapsed: he was vomiting again and had diarrhea and fever. Again, she tried herbal medicine of bark and leaves. First, she tried one type, but it did not help; then she used the *Sambnoré* again, both to purge the child and to wash him. She also bought a few tablets of Nivaquine and APC (malaria medicine) from the market. She had consulted neither Dr. Sorgho nor the dispensary due to lack of money, explaining: "It is a problem of money, if I go to Dr. Sorgho, or at Tenga [the dispensary] twice, there is no money left to take him the next time." At the fifth week's visit, Kabiro was still vomiting and had diarrhea after each meal. His navel was swollen and hot. Based on advice from a local healer, his mother had not purged him for three days. After giving him two tablets of malaria medicine, she again consulted the local healer, who treated the child's navel; she told me, they would be visiting this healer for a third time the coming Monday. She would have to leave early, she explained, as the treatment needed to take place before the child ate anything.

I accompanied Kabiro and his mother to the local healer for their consultation. We walked over to the healer's compound, situated only ten minutes from the house of Kabiro's family. The compounds were connected by small paths that crisscross the village area. Just before the harvest, it is sometimes difficult to find the tracks, as millet and maize are grown in small plots between the compounds. The compound of this healer was, like most other compounds, surrounded by a high mud wall. In recent years, many of the mud walls have been replaced by brick walls plastered with mud. Such walls are more robust and do not break down as easily in the heavy rains. At the healer's compound, an elderly woman was waiting, sitting on a small wooden stool in front of her house. She seemed to know what she was doing and appeared confident about her treatment. The healer had a small box containing a black powder and some very hot water. She lifted Kabiro up and placed him over her knees with his stomach down, holding him firmly. He was definitely not happy about being placed in this position. While the healer held the crying child on her knees, his mother took the small open box up to his navel and held it there for about ten minutes. She then removed the box again at the instruction of the healer, and a small black piece of "gum" was found in the box. They took it out and showed it to me. "This is the disease," the healer announced; it had been expelled from the navel, they explained. Then, the mother took the box outside the compound and threw the contents away. This was the third and last treatment of this kind, and both mother and healer said that the piece of gum was smaller this time. After the treatment, this specific disease, *puga* (stomach), would never attack the child again. According to convention, boys needed to undergo this treatment three times while girls needed the treatment four times (Fainzang 1985b, 1986).[9]

Juggling Multiple Pathways

In Keru, mothers' pathways to find healing for their children were seldom linear. Worried about the potential cost of treatment, they often tried the least expensive avenues first. Before consulting any specialist, they often departed for the bush to find specific leaves, roots, or bark, which they brought home and prepared for the treatment of a sick child. Alternatively, they bought allopathic medicine at the local market, where products were often sold by the piece. It was considered an advantage that pharmaceuticals often were sold in small quantities; buying just a couple of pills made it possible to evaluate whether the medicine actually reduced the symptoms without having to buy the full course of treatment. As documented in other studies on treatment-seeking practices (Colvin et al. 2013; Müller et al. 2003; Olsen and Sargent 2017; Østergaard, Bjertrup, and Samuelsen 2016; Samuelsen 2004b), mothers' responses to child illness can be divided into three forms of action: (1) home treatment with herbal medicine or pharmaceuticals bought from the local market, (2) consultation with traditional healers or persons with particular insights, and (3) consultation with a biomedical specialist within the public health care system, usually the rural dispensary.

Mothers with sick children did not have the privilege of developing complete strategies. Instead, they had to "make do," taking one step at a time, reflecting on the situation, and looking for available and affordable therapeutic pathways. While some pathways close, others open, giving space for agency and hope. The health care-seeking trajectories, the therapeutic as well as preventive activities such as vaccinating children and buying amulets, were to large extent about juggling the possibilities of the moment. Thus, it was not necessarily contradictory to consult both the public health care facilities and so-called traditional healers. Searching out different treatment options is about taking advantage of available opportunities. Moving from one health care service to another should not necessarily be interpreted as a strategic choice between medical systems or specific epistemologies, but rather as a responsible way of maneuvering in a complex field of potentialities, where propitious moments are seized (Hänsch et al. 2017). Mothers based their choice of therapy on past experiences, as well as on a range of other pragmatic issues such as availability, distance, cost, and time, as we will see in Fati's case below.

Fati was the mother of Zakaria, a three-year-old child who had been sick for almost three weeks when I met them in 2010. He was suffering from fever and diarrhea, and he had an infected abscess on his left eyelid. This was not the first time he had gotten an infection there, so now Fati massaged the eyelid with shea butter and gave him half a tablet of aspirin, morning and evening. On previous occasions, she had consulted both the dispensary and Dr. Sorgho's private clinic, explaining to me that this time, "Dr. Sorgho is tired of treating us. We now leave it in the hands of God." According to Fati, this disease affected her son during the rainy season, when the trees caused abscesses. Over a couple of weeks, Fati continued to massage the abscess with shea butter and rinse it with *gohini*, a powder made from a local tree. After three weeks Zakaria was better, but only a few days after that the illness returned: "The illness is back again, it starts all over again with diarrhea, fever and the infected abscess—it is the third time like this." Again, she started treatment by massaging the eyelid with shea butter and gave him a biomedical product. She did not remember its name, as she bought it from a woman in the compound who sold various pharmaceuticals. She had purchased three tablets and gave them to her son over three days.

Fati was the wife of the *delegué* (village representative) and lived in a huge family compound, including several generations and many brothers and uncles with their wives and children. There were many women within the household with whom to share experiences and from whom Fati received advice about how to treat Zakaria's sickness. For Fati, the abscess was the real problem, and the diarrhea and fever were additional symptoms of this sickness. She was clearly concerned about the recurrent abscess as well as her son's health more generally, complaining that he continued to nurse although he was almost four years old and she had no more milk. This is not normal, she said, as her other children stopped breastfeeding after about one year because she stopped producing milk. Zakaria was weakened by the recurrent sickness, and Fati was exhausted after providing ongoing care. After another couple of weeks, she decided to consult Dr. Sorgho again.

Zakaria's course of sickness and Fati's course of action are in many ways typical. Zakaria was suffering from a number of symptoms, which could be related but could instead be symptoms of more than one disease. The diagnosis was unclear, and the symptoms continued for a long time, waning for short periods only to reappear again and again. Suffering from diarrhea, fever, and an infected abscess for months weakened Zakaria. In this way, his experience was typical, as many children in this area were weakened from recurrent diseases, often in combination with malnutrition. Fati's many efforts to heal Zakaria are also typical: starting with some herbal treatment at home, buying a few medical products at the market, and changing the course of treatment over time in the hope that these low-cost therapies will work. As in Kabiro's case, biomedicine as well as several different types of herbal medicines (such as bark and leaves) were used at different moments during Zakaria's illness. The biomedical treatments from the pensioned nurse, Dr. Sorgho, and at the rural dispensary were for malaria. None of these treatments seemed to cure the boy. Perhaps he actually suffered from malaria, but it could be that he also suffered from one or more other diseases. Such comorbidities are probably very common but are difficult for the dispensary staff to diagnose due to lack of equipment. The mother also tried to treat him with malaria medicine herself, but she was not following a dosage regime; instead, she dissolved a few tablets and purged him.

In this part of Burkina Faso, all mothers with sick children were painfully aware of the cost of treatment; the widespread practice of home treatment had to do with keeping costs down. Uncertainties about the cost for treatment at the dispensary, even in periods where treatment of children under five is, in principle, free, lead many women to refrain from choosing public health care facilities as the first option. Mothers of sick children and ill adults often explain that they have not consulted the primary health care center because "Il n'y a pas d'argent" (there is no money). As Zenabo, an elderly woman living in the village of Bangri, said with a sense of irony: "You want to go there, but when you have no money . . . if you went to the hospital [dispensary] every day, would they give you the products as a gift?" Safi Aminata, a staff member at the local dispensary, confirmed that home treatment was the first option for many people, saying: "When we receive a sick person here, and we ask when the illness started, they often respond that it started fifteen days ago, or more than two weeks ago. When we then ask why she had not consulted us at the dispensary, she says that they treat at home first with local products or medicines bought at the market—and when they see no improvements, they prefer our services. It is very difficult for us to know which products they have used." Therapeutic pathways in Burkina Faso and other parts of the world often zigzag between therapeutic options, particularly in complex or prolonged illness (Foley 2009; Mogensen 2005; Olsen and Sargent 2017; Whyte 1997). The strategy of starting with home treatment before turning to other options has not changed much over the years. However, data from the Demographic Health Surveys and my own observations suggest that the demand for public health care services is increasing.

The Chronicity of Everyday Emergencies

As I talked with mothers about recent episodes of illness among their children, they often mentioned the word *yingwingre*, which literally means "warm body." Of fifty interviews with mothers about recent child illness, thirty-seven responded that they had experienced illness among their children during the previous two weeks. Most of the episodes concerned children under five years old, and in nineteen cases the illness was labeled *yinwingre*. The translation of *yinwingre* in the Mossi-French dictionary is "fievre, palu" (fever, malaria). The mothers themselves did not necessarily identify this disease as malaria; rather, it was a description of the symptoms: the body of the child was warm. Many mothers saw this illness caused by the child being excessively exposed to heat or to the strong sun, not necessarily to mosquito bites.

As the mothers respond to illness, they act in a kind of "subjunctive mode," hoping for the best and keeping all options open (Whyte 1997). They find themselves in a permanently acute situation. Their small children often fall sick, and while relapses are common, their immediate goal is to bring relief to the child. Child sickness in rural Burkina Faso is in this sense endemic rather than episodic. During the actual episode of illness, the outcome is always uncertain. Caregivers were less concerned about the specific cause of the disease than about finding solutions and exploring alternative treatment options (Østergaard et al. 2016). They managed uncertainty by working with a maximum of possibilities and juggling various options, while at the same time being pragmatic and constantly worrying about how to pay for the next treatment. During early childhood, sickness is part of everyday life (and death); the child falls sick, gets better, then soon relapses. The chronicity of childhood illness is characterized by an unpredictable series of infectious diseases and comorbidities demanding action every time the child falls ill. In each case of sickness, every deterioration generates new worries and uncertainties. It is a chronicity characterized by everyday emergencies (Manderson and Warren 2016; Millar 2014; Vigh 2008).

Conclusion

I have in this chapter described the everyday care work mothers engaged in, with an emphasis on how demanding, intense, and time-consuming it is to ensure the survival of small children born in this part of the world. Small children continue to be in relationship with the spiritual world during their first years of life, and their small bodies are susceptible to a range of illnesses, many of which are not easy to cure. Children in Keru suffered from recurrent illnesses, with fever and stomach problems the most commonly reported symptoms. Despite their mothers' diligent care, children were rarely cured before the next disease attacked or the same disease returned. The mothers were attentive to their children's needs and took responsibility to provide appropriate care. Most cases of illness were open to a diverse range of interpretations, making it more difficult to ascertain the most appropriate treatment at the time of the outbreak and throughout the period of illness. Each step in the therapeutic process was loaded with uncertainties and ambiguities. For mothers in Keru, the public health care system did not emerge as an unremitting safety net in cases of child sickness. Mothers' hopes were not exclusively invested in the knowledge and skills of the professional health care staff at the local dispensary or nearby hospital, but in pragmatic pathways combining home treatment, consultations with traditional healers, and visits to the pensioned nurse. Mothers sought to protect their children, preventing diseases and other dangers and taking action when children fell ill. Both caring and illness are relational, as we saw in the case of the sudden death of Caro's child, where marital problems and accusations of witchcraft were interpreted as causing the death of the child.

Notes

Epigraph: Okri (1991) 1993: 3.

1. According to Caro, the mother-in-law converted from Islam to Christianity some years back; however, she continued to support her son's position that the child should be brought up within the father's religion, which in this case is Islam.
2. This is the direct quote in French. Whether the mother-in-law actually consumed the fetishes, or whether Caro used the term *bouffer* as a description of the act of sacrifice is unclear.
3. UNICEF, "The State of the World's Children 2021." Retrieved 15 July 2023 from https://www.unicef.org/reports/state-worlds-children-2021.
4. See chapter 1 for a more elaborate description of Jean and his role in the village.
5. See also Samuelsen (1998) for a description of this case.
6. *Zugu* literally means "head." It is an expression used for this sickness of the fontanel, but it is also used to describe headache and other illnesses affecting the head.
7. The Benjamin is an expression used to describe the youngest child in a family referring to the biblical story of Jacob and his wife Rachel, Benjamin was their youngest child.
8. The case of Kabiro was observed in 1997; however, in more recent studies in the same area, we find similar patterns.

9. In large parts of West Africa, it is common to ascribe the number three to males and the number four to females. Symbolic interpretations often relate to the male and female anatomy. Sylvie Fainzang (1985a) suggests that the discourse implied by this symbolism serves to establish social relations between the sexes and to legitimize male domination.

Chapter 3
Migration as Care Work

Michel looked smart and stylish as he sat casually on a chair wearing jeans, a short black leather jacket, and a huge wristwatch. Janine, his younger sister, showed me proudly the photo of Michel in February 2020. We sat for a long time looking at the photo, commenting on all the details, and we both agreed he seemed to have developed into a good-looking and trendy young man.

More than six years had passed since I last saw Michel in Keru before he embarked on his *aventure*, yet he was easy to recognize. He now looked more mature than the teenager I had last seen in the village. Michel had left the village back in 2014 in order to try his luck as a migrant worker in Libya. Long before he left for Libya, he and his family had discussed the possibilities he had for sustaining himself and supporting his family. As a child, he had never been eager to go to school, and, despite Thomas and Beatrice encouraging all of their children to continue their education, he left after primary level (six years of schooling). After his early teenage years, when he had helped his father and older brother Pascal in the fields and hung around in the village with a group of other teenagers, the family persuaded him to attend a vocational training center in the nearby town. He was not sure about which profession he would go for, as he did not have a devotion to any specific field. He decided that he would start training as electrician because both he and the family were convinced that it would be easy to find a job as soon as he finished. However, he soon realized that this particular program was rather theoretical, so he got permission from the director of the school to switch to a program in auto mechanics. The vocational training center was new and well equipped. The director, who had received engineering training in Germany, was very enthusiastic and wanted to ensure that the young people at the training center would eventually work as hard and be as disciplined as the workers he had encountered in Germany. The center had been funded by the government of Taiwan, and it offered a range of vocational training programs for both men and women, including theoretical and practical classes ranging from carpentry to tailoring. The workshops were all well equipped except for the auto shop, which was still short of equipment. The trainees had to pay for their own safety shoes and uniforms, as well as a yearly school fee. Thomas had arranged for Michel to stay with family members in town on weekdays to minimize his transportation costs. It was a two-year program, but for various reasons Michel quit the school after some months and returned home. It was around that time that the family discussions about Michel's possibilities for "taking his turn" as a migrant worker intensified.

After some considerations, they decided that Michel should leave for Guinea to find work. The family had some contacts there through other members of the Keru community that they planned to use in order to find accommodations and facilitate his job search. However, in 2014, the borders between Burkina Faso and a number of West African countries closed due to the Ebola epidemic in Liberia, Guinea, and Sierra Leone. At that time, it was unclear when borders would open again; hence, after serious consideration, the family decided that Michel, like many other West African young people, should head north to seek work. The family mobilized a rather large sum of money to secure his transport through the Sahara Desert to reach Libya. Six years later, Michel was still there. Although the photo of Michel exposed a young man shining with self-confidence, it was also clear from the limited information the family received from him that the years in Libya had been tough. His family in Keru was unsure about how much work he had, where he lived, or how his social life had developed. He did not reveal a lot when they occasionally spoke over the phone. Perhaps he talked more confidentially with his brother Pascal, but the rest of the family did not know much about his daily challenges. After six years, the family was eager for him to return to Burkina Faso, not least because of Thomas's increasingly frail health. Michel had also indicated that he wanted to come home, but, as I describe below, he had not yet been in a position to leave Libya.

Migration as Care Work

In Keru, most families depend on long-distance social relations as many villagers, mostly young men, migrate to other countries to look for work. This is not a new phenomenon. The plantation economy in Côte d'Ivoire has for decades been an important destination for labor migrants from Burkina Faso. During the French colonization of West Africa, the present-day territories of Burkina Faso and Côte d'Ivoire were tightly linked, with Burkina Faso serving as a labor reserve and Côte d'Ivoire as the location of a lucrative plantation economy that continues to be important today (Bjarnesen 2013: 17; Cross 2020; Kleist and Bjarnesen 2019). However, West Africa has been and continues to be characterized by political instability and armed conflict. Political conflicts in Côte d'Ivoire have disrupted cross-border migration from Burkina Faso on several occasions. In the 1990s, internal political conflicts between politicians of the north and politicians of the south in Côte d'Ivoire instigated a nationalist discourse with radical definitions of *Ivorité* (Ivorianness) and severe public hostility against non-Ivorian civilians (Bjarnesen 2013; Mitchell 2012). During the autumn of 1999, this controversy resulted in violent conflicts and forced the evacuation of more than ten thousand Burkinabes from southwest Côte d'Ivoire. The so-called autochthony discourses continued after the 2010 elections in Côte d'Ivoire with numerous violent episodes in the western cocoa regions where many Burkinabe migrants work. The continued political conflicts in Côte d'Ivoire contribute to further uncertainties for Burkinabe citizens, in terms of both job opportunities and security.

For many, both the individuals who migrate as well as the families staying behind, the migration period is difficult. Some of the migrants, like Michel, embark on high-risk journeys through the Sahara Desert, and a few travel even further, crossing the Mediterranean Sea to Europe. The majority of the migrants from Keru are young men who have to rely on the mercy of the human intermediaries they pay to guide them through the dangerous terrain. The family members staying behind continue their everyday lives, looking forward to news from their relatives and hoping that their young family representatives will be able to send money home.

In this chapter, I argue that labor migration should be seen in a wider context of social relations and social obligations. It is not only about striving for material gains beyond subsistence agriculture; it is also about *care labor*, to use Hannah Arendt's distinction between work and labor. Drawing on John Locke's distinction between working hands and a laboring body, Arendt emphasizes three fundamental forms of human activity: labor, work, and action.[1] I am here particularly interested in Arendt's focus on labor as everyday work, "the monotonous performance of daily repeated chores" (Arendt 2013: 100), which, I argue, also includes activities related to the sustenance of one's family and kin. Michel and Pascal both left the village to seek work in order to support and care for their family back home and to secure a future for themselves and the next generation. Their cases illustrate the importance of *work*, understood both as an economic activity and as *care labor*, the obligation to support family and kin (Alber and Drotbohm 2015). Erdmute Alber and Heike Drotbohm contend that "emigration and assumptions of upward economic mobility will provide the migrant with the capacity to care" (2015: 8). Thus, migration as a form of "transnational care" is not only about sending remittances but also about nurturing kinship relations.

After analyzing out-migration as care labor, I then switch focus to the many wives "staying behind" in the village, waiting for remittances and a successful husband to return home. To a certain extent, they become even more immobilized. They become physically immobile, as they have long days farming the land and taking care of the children, reducing their possibilities for further education or training. Socially, they find themselves in a stand-by position, waiting for remittances or their husband's return with financial capital. At the same time, some of the women take advantage of their responsibility for the household by finding new ways of generating income and by organizing themselves in various women's groups. While many couples have little contact during the often yearlong migration periods, the husbands remain important "absent-present" figures within the households. The sporadic contact many wives have with their absent husbands exposes them to a number of uncertainties, including uncertainties about how to manage the next meal, how to deal with illness, and how to negotiate their position in the household of the absent husband's family. Migration and remittances play a vital role in the local economy in this part of Burkina Faso, and they shape local care activities in gendered ways.

According to the village chief, almost all households in Keru include at least one member who temporarily works outside of the village. Demographic pressures on the land and increasingly unstable seasonal rains (probably due to climate change; see Alvar-Beltrán et al. 2020) make it unsustainable for the younger generations to make a living from subsistence farming, small-scale gardening, and husbandry alone. Burkina Faso is ranked seventh among the top twenty countries experiencing migration—almost 8 percent of its population has emigrated. UNICEF estimated that in 2013 about 1.6 million Burkinabes of a total population of around 16 million had emigrated, with Côte d'Ivoire the destination for 1.4 million of the migrants (Awumbila 2018).[2] Drawing on data in 2003 from four Burkinabe villages, Fleur Wouterse found that 62 percent of all households had one or more migrants who were away for more than one month per year, most of whom were young men with little education (Wouterse 2010). That profile matches that of many migrants from Keru, including Michel and Pascal.[3]

Going on *Aventure*

In Keru, migrants are said to go on *aventure* (adventure) when they leave the village in order to find work outside of Burkina Faso, whether they are heading to other West or Central African countries such as Côte d'Ivoire, Gabon, Guinea, or Ghana or are traveling north across the Sahara Desert to Libya or Europe. To "go on *aventure*" alludes to a journey that may be exciting but also dangerous. It is my impression from conversations with young men in Keru that they are very aware of this double meaning of the term and express their full commitment to both the exciting and risky parts of the journey. As Catherine Conrad Suso discusses, out-migration in contemporary Africa is often seen as a *rite de passage*, a way to mature and gain knowledge about the world (Conrad Suso 2020).

Many young people in Keru are eager to move away from the village. They know that their chance of prospering as a rural farmer is limited, not least because of the land inheritance system in which farmland is divided among the sons who are staying in the village. Thomas, Michel's father, inherited half of the family land from his father while his brother got the other half. If Thomas's two sons were to inherit the fields in the same way, they would each get a quarter of the land that their grandfather had. They both know this is unsustainable; one of them has to leave or find additional income substantial enough to sustain his own family. For most of the residents of Keru, migrant work is seen as an "experience of continual return," not as an end in itself (Millar 2014; Schapendonk, Bolay, and Dahinden 2020). Migrants hope to visit home once or twice each year, or alternate a couple of years abroad with a couple of years at home. The dream for most migrants and their families is to find a stable, long-term job abroad that would allow them to send enough money home to support the family in their everyday life and in cases of sickness. They also hope to save money to construct a better house for themselves and their family upon their return (Alber and Drotbohm 2015; Kleist and Jansen 2016; Lucht 2011). For decades, migration has served as a practical way for young people to respond to the expectations and familial pressure to generate an income and take care of their relatives, obligations that are otherwise difficult to honor because of economic decline, land pressure, and climate change. Both young men and young women are concerned about their fragile prospects for a successful future. For women, who often have only a few years of schooling, marriage has traditionally been the most viable option to secure their own future and relieve their parents from having to support them beyond childhood. For many young men, facing the chronic economic crisis in Burkina Faso with few opportunities to get a job, it has become increasingly difficult to attain a traditional masculine position in society. The patriarchal and virilocal system, which obligates male community members to sustain the well-being of relatives and honor family relations, continues to be extremely important, as documented in other West African ethnographies (Bjarnesen 2013; Lucht 2011; Vigh 2017). To provide relational care involves both "labor" and "work," using Arendt's distinction, where "work" refers primarily to the production of finished products and "labor" relates to the daily chores characteristic of the private household or farm (Arendt 2013). In chapter 2, I discussed work and care labor in relation to the obligations that wives and mothers have toward their families and kin. Here, I argue that labor migration is another form of care labor.

In his introduction to *Ordinary Ethics*, Michael Lambek emphasized the importance of *care*, saying, "Care signifies, in the first instance, looking after, or looking out for, the well-being of others, and

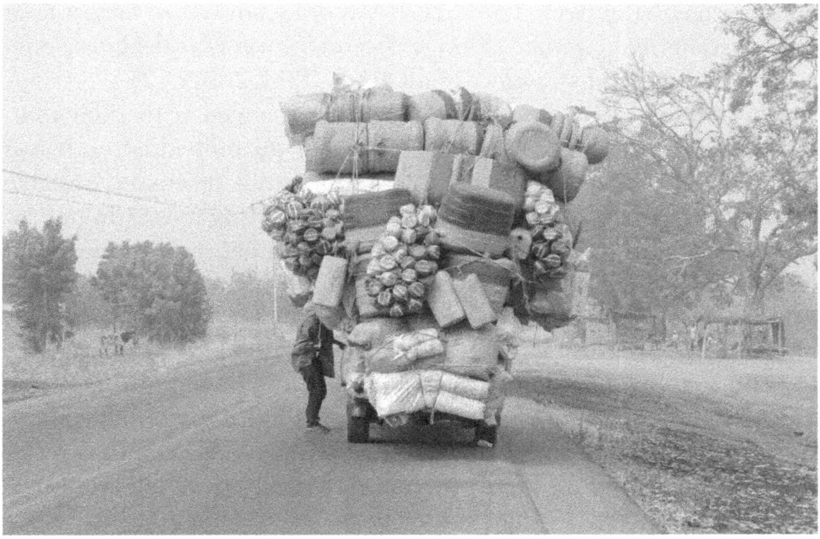

Figure 3.1. Loaded van, Burkina Faso (© Helle Samuelsen 2023)

as such it both is central to what anthropologists have constructed as the domain of kinship and serves to remind us that kinship is fundamentally a realm of ethical activity" (Lambek 2010: 15). When residents of Keru take risks to seek work far away, they do so as part of a life-course transition, as a move toward maturity, independence, and income generation, but also as part of their obligation to provide a safe and secure future for close family and kin. They may put their own life and health at risk, but the journey serves a vital purpose. Being aware of both their purposes and their sacrifices, they affirm who they are in relation to others (Alber and Drotbohm 2015; Van Nistelrooy 2014: 520). This kind of social obligation links to Paul Ricoeur's point about the intrinsic relationship between fragility and responsibility. In his reflections on the fundamental human dependency of self and other, Ricoeur says, "The selfhood of oneself implies otherness to such an intimate degree that one cannot be thought of without the other" (1994: 3). In the philosophy of the Danish theologian Knud Ejler Løgstrup, we find a similar definition of the individual as first and foremost a dependent and relational being: "An unspoken demand lies in any kind of meeting between human beings independent of the circumstances and character the meeting has" (Løgstrup 1991: 26).[4] We are who we are by virtue of our relations to parents, siblings, friends, lovers, colleagues, enemies, children, and strangers of all kinds (Fink 2007: 12).

The migrating youth are intrinsically entangled with their families; for most of them, the journey is not an individual endeavor but a family project. In Michel's case, the family discussed possible destinations and made the travel possible by saving money to pay for the journey and his initial stay in Libya. The decision to move out of the village for an unknown period of time to find work is a moral act, an attempt to live up to one's obligations (and the expectations of relatives). Neither Michel nor his family understood themselves to be in a completely desperate situation before he left. Although for most people in rural Burkina Faso life is full of uncertainties about the next harvest and the outcome of the next case of malaria or other illness, Michel and his family had lived through those uncertainties. Some years the harvest had been abundant, other years it had been meager, but they had managed. However, at the time of Michel's departure in 2014, the family, particularly Thomas and Beatrice, were facing a fragile future. Their elder son was supposed to take over from Thomas as head of household and take responsibility for farming their land. However, he was still not married, and his *aventure* to Côte d'Ivoire had been unsuccessful because of a serious injury that continued to cause problems. Michel, their other son, had to find a path that would support himself and his own future family—and hopefully also support his parents when they were no longer able to work. High unemployment rates among young people in the major cities of Burkina Faso and a looming political crisis diminished the prospects for young people with little schooling like Michel.

In the conclusion to his book about Ghanaian migrants in Naples, Italy, Hans Lucht asked rhetorically: "But why do the migrants risk their lives by coming to Europe, and why do they choose to substitute their friends and families at home with such a difficult and even hostile environment?" Lucht provides the answer himself, saying:

> Viewing high-risk migration as either a matter of obtaining material gains or the result of sheer thoughtlessness, with all its biased connotations, is not a satisfactory explanation. To be sure, material gains often articulate social and existential needs, but these needs cannot be reduced to the gains themselves. Moreover, the Guan migrants have relatively deep knowledge about the dangers and hardships of the journey at the

> time they decide to take their chances, suggesting that they knowingly put their lives at risk and willingly endure the hardships of migrant life in Naples—because they feel they have no other options. (Lucht 2011: 263)

This conclusion also applies to migrants from Keru, whether they cross the borders to neighboring countries to find work or they embark on the high-risk journey through the Sahara Desert to Libya (with few of them traveling onward to Europe). Being photographed with a nice leather jacket and a large wristwatch gave Michel an opportunity to expose his material "wealth." However, his family was fully aware that he was a proud man who did not want to return home empty-handed. This was one of the reasons his *aventure* in Libya had lasted more than six years. For the migrants, the "adventure" no doubt entails dreams about jobs, material goods, and not least the ability to send remittances home, but the decision is also based on deep knowledge about the risks, sacrifices, and tough living and working conditions they will face.

Missing Documents

Michel did find temporary jobs in Libya, mostly short-term positions as a day laborer in plumbing or construction. It was, however, difficult to decipher how much work he actually had. When Janine and I looked at the photo in 2020, he had assured his sister that his accommodations were acceptable, but she did not know much about his daily life or living conditions. The family knew, however, that Michel had converted to Islam. Janine told me this while we looked at his photo, noting that Michel had to pray on Fridays. I was surprised by the news because the family, as previously mentioned, was active in the local Catholic mission, where Thomas had served for many years as catechist. Janine smiled and said that her mother, before marrying Thomas, used to be called Binta, as she used to be a Muslim. Curious, I asked how Thomas had reacted to Michel's conversion. Janine replied: "Well, you know my father is not very strict. He does not prevent us from that; he is a democrat!"

Several times since 2015, the International Organization for Migration (IOM) has, in collaboration with the embassy of Burkina Faso, organized voluntary repatriation flights from Libya to Burkina Faso for illegal Burkinabe immigrants. In 2016, when many migrants trying to cross the Mediterranean were dying, a total of 160 migrants were repatriated back to Burkina Faso.[5] Similar flights were organized in the following years. In 2016, Michel had indicated to his family that he would like to return home, as it was difficult to find work. According to his father, Michel had been offered the possibility of repatriation but had declined. To him, it would be shameful to be repatriated, as it would indicate that he had been unable to pay for his own ticket and would expose his lack of economic success. In 2020, Janine said with a sad smile as she looked at the photo of Michel on her phone: "Every time we call him, we ask him to come home because we really need him now. It has been a long time and we miss him. We really miss him." Before he left for Libya, he got engaged to a girl from one of the neighboring villages. The girl continued to wait for him to come home, as Janine explained: "Oh, you know, here, with us, it is like that; the rigidity of the parents makes it impossible to escape, you cannot leave your boyfriend or girlfriend like that, unless there are serious problems between you—then the parents may authorize you to split, but if the in-laws first have received the kola nuts, you cannot split up."[6] The girlfriend had to wait for him to return to Burkina.

Again, in 2020, Michel had talked about returning home, but he did not possess a national identity card documenting that he was a Burkinabe citizen. According to Janine, he had tried twice to apply for the CNIB (Carte Nationale d'Identité Burkinabé) in 2014 before leaving for Libya; however, the card had not been issued by the authorities. Janine explained:

> He had applied for it twice. He went to Ouaga and applied, but it was not issued. After that, he went to Tenkodogo, and the same thing happened, so he left like that. Illegally, he entered illegally. Now, in order to return, he again has to travel illegally, but as the countries [he has to pass through] are not secure, it is a bit complicated. He has asked me to send him his birth certificate in order to get a passport issued. Then he would return by air. He has given me a telephone number to a person working at the embassy of Burkina in Libya, who currently should be here in Ouaga. He asked me to give the birth certificate to that person who could bring it to Libya in order for him to get a passport issued. But it has not been possible for me to get in contact with this person, so I really don't know what to do. But I have asked him if it would be possible for him to return home with a "laisser-passer," as it is said that if you don't have a passport

> you can return if you have a "laisser-passer." But I don't know if this is possible for him. I really don't know.

Michel was, in other words, not able to prove his identity as a citizen of Burkina Faso without an identity card. He had left the country illegally without an identity card and was now barred from crossing borders legally in order to return to Burkina Faso. The state had suddenly surfaced as an important player in Michel's life. Before he left for Libya, he had experienced the arbitrariness of state bureaucratic procedures when, for some reason, he was unsuccessful in getting a national identity card. As a result, Michel found himself in a kind of limbo. He was determined to return home, but he could not prove his identity and therefore worried about embarking on another high-risk journey through the Sahara Desert and a number of insecure countries. When crossing the borders—the margins of the state—the otherwise "absent" state becomes visible, with the power to include or exclude individuals (Das and Poole 2004; Ferme 2004; Heyman and Symons 2012).

In addition, Michel's many years in Libya had not been the economic success he and his family had hoped. He had not been able to save much and only occasionally sent remittances home. Another young man from Keru who had left for Libya together with Michel had returned home after a couple of years. He had been in Libya with his wife and a small child, but they had decided to return because it was too difficult for him to find sufficient work. In the village, his decision to return home and his admission that it had been difficult to find a job to support his family were seen as brave, but he himself did not talk much about his experiences in Libya.

Michel and his family had saved money for his journey to Libya, which they all knew would be a high-risk *aventure*. After Pascal's unsuccessful migration experience in Côte d'Ivoire, the pressure on Michel was high. In Keru, the households with successful migrants are easy to identify because of their larger two- or three-room square houses with corrugated roofs. The family back home worried a lot, and they also realized that Michel's stay in Libya dragged on both because he felt he needed to engage in *care labor* by finding work and saving money, and because his return was complicated by "paperwork" problems.

Immobilities and Invisibilities

Migration is often viewed optimistically for its potential to generate household income and to spur development, while the unseen costs to those staying behind are often ignored. As Torres emphasizes: "It is often the 'immobile' who are most affected by migration, with the heaviest burdens falling on the women, children, elderly, sick and disabled who remain behind in origin communities" (Torres 2015: 365). In this section, I will zoom in on another aspect of care labor related to the out-migration of so many young people, mostly men, from Keru. The migrants often stay away for years while their wives remain in the village with a huge amount of care labor to carry out.[7] I argue that many women staying behind live in a fragile state of *triple uncertainty*. First, like other rural citizens, they live with the uncertainties regarding the possible outcome of the next harvest. Second, like many other families in Keru, they face uncertainties related to the high frequency of sickness among their children. The difference for the mothers staying behind, though, is that their husbands are not around to support them in caring for the children. Third, they live with uncertainties about when and how much they will receive in remittances from their husbands and when their husbands will return home (Mikal et al. 2020). While the majority of the wives staying behind were affected by the hardship of taking care of the farmland and the family during their husband's absence, a few managed to explore the opportunities of being the de facto head of household.

More than forty years ago, Esther Boserup focused specifically on African women's huge contribution to agricultural production, both during and after the colonial period, pointing out that much of this work was invisible in the statistics (Boserup 1970, 1980). Until Boserup's pioneering book *Woman's Role in Economic Development*, the specific role of women in production had been largely ignored in the scientific literature on development issues. Although a number of anthropologists had dealt with the role of women in a changing society, Boserup's work was groundbreaking because it was the first in-depth analysis of women's economic contributions. She argued that women's heavy involvement in food cultivation, particularly in Africa, generated a pattern of predominantly male migration, leaving women and children in the village (Beneria and Sen 1981). I do not argue here that the family members staying behind necessarily bear the heaviest burden, but I argue that many of the wives remaining in the village are left with a huge amount of care labor, placing them in an extremely fragile context of multiple uncertainties.

In the village of Keru, the vast majority of women are active in agricultural production. Besides working in the family fields, women are often allotted a piece of land by their husbands to grow millet, sorghum, maize, or other products for household consumption. If they grow cash crops or vegetables in a separate garden, they have the possibility of controlling the income themselves, as husbands and wives have separate economies in this part of Burkina Faso. Conversations with women in Keru who are "staying behind" demonstrate that they contribute care labor that includes agricultural work on their own plots of lands and on their husband's or family's fields in addition to the traditional household activities of cooking and childcare.

For five years, Claire had been living in her in-laws' compound with two children, six and nine years of age, while her husband was in Gabon. During the first three years, according to Claire, her husband had a good job and had been able to send money home for the reconstruction of their house. He used to regularly send 10,000 CFA [franc] (US$18.00) or 20,000 CFA [franc] (US$36.00), "but during the last two years until today, it is not going well."[8] The husband left the village when the youngest child was only nine months old and had not been back since. He called regularly to ask how they were doing at home, and she sent him photos of the children via mobile phone. Their youngest child had not yet started school despite being old enough. Since birth he had suffered from anemia and often fell ill. Every time he fell ill, Claire went to the dispensary in Keru where the nurse prescribed a blood transfusion. She then went to the regional hospital to buy a bag of blood for the transfusion. Claire depended on the irregular remittances from her husband to pay for this treatment.

The family compound where she was living included Claire and her children, her parents-in-law, and her brothers-in-law and their wives and children. Claire farmed her husband's land, growing red sorghum, rice, maize, and beans for herself and her children, saying: "It is only for consumption. If the harvest is not sufficient to feed the family, you cannot sell anything. We do not do large-scale farming; it is only in small quantity. We farm to have something to eat." Claire's story illustrates how the everyday life of the wives staying behind is characterized by uncertainties. In addition to the uncertainties about subsistence agriculture and illness, she did not know when her husband would send her money or when he intended to return home. In the meantime, she depended on her in-laws if she had expenses she could not cover herself. Assana, whose husband was in Côte d'Ivoire, expressed her frustration and uncertainty in the following way: "Sometimes, the harvest is poor. All the children are our responsibility. The 10,000 CFA [franc] [US$18.00] cannot cover our needs. We have to rely on the 10,000 CFA [franc] to buy soap and shoes. It is really difficult."

Laurentine was one of the few women I met in Keru who had left the village with her husband to find work. She spent almost seven years in Equatorial Guinea from 2009 to 2016, interrupted only by one year back in Keru in 2012. After 2016, she stayed in Keru while her husband worked with a construction crew on the main road from Burkina to Togo. They had been able to construct new houses for themselves and other family members and to save some money for the future education of their children. Now, she wanted to stay in the village, saying, "We want to stay here because life is not easy in Equatorial Guinea. If you leave without papers in order to find work, you will not be able to work. And it is very expensive to get the papers organized in Guinea. Thus, it is not easy to work there. Often you might work but not receive all your salary. That's why we have returned home. Some of our money we didn't even get with us." She continued describing her experience in Guinea:

> The health and the police were our biggest problems there. You are not able to save money as you should. In Equatorial Guinea, if you don't have at least 50,000 CFA [franc], you cannot get your papers issued. If you earn 150,000 CFA [franc] a month, how will you then save money, when you also have to get food and pay for health care? Then it is better to return to your home. The biggest problem was the police who took our money. Before going to hospital, you have to pay the police, even though you have your papers. When you then arrive, they ask: "Who are you?" If you then say that you are Burkinabe or from Côte d'Ivoire, even if you show your papers, you have to pay 2,000 CFA [franc] before leaving the hospital.

When I asked Laurentine what made them decide to migrate in 2009, she replied: "You can see the situation yourself. Here, there

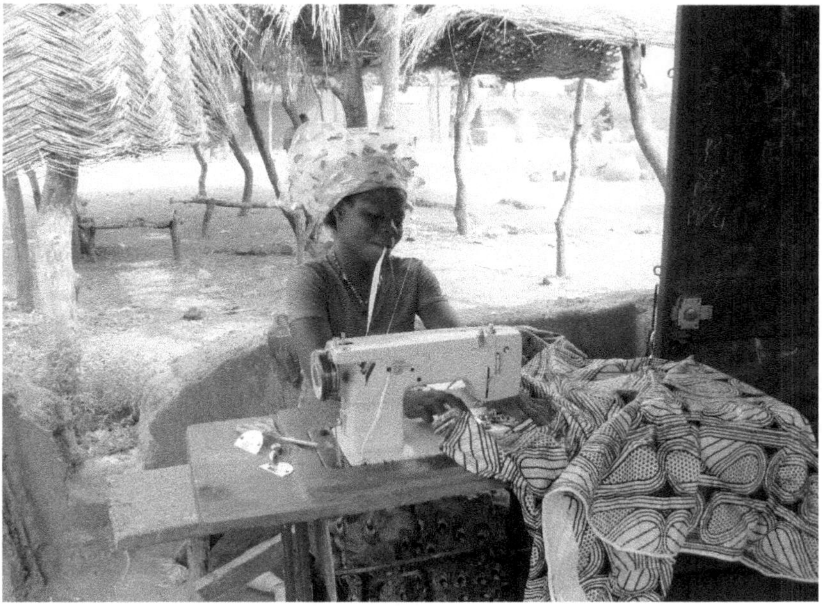

Figure 3.2. Female tailor, rural Burkina Faso (© Helle Samuelsen 2023)

are no jobs. If you stay here with your family and the rains are not plentiful, there is not enough food. What can you do in such a situation? The children are there. The family is also there. Also, in order to get a nice house, you cannot continue to sleep."

Many women whose husbands were away showed abundant agency, energy, and creativity in generating supplementary income. Besides tending their own fields and their husband's fields, some grew vegetables such as tomatoes and onions in vegetable gardens. Some produced food to sell in small restaurants on market days, and others bought bread in nearby towns to sell in the village. I met Mouna at the marketplace in Keru on her way home after having sold Ghanaian bread at the market.[9] Mouna was talkative and did not seem shy, as many other female residents in rural Burkina Faso do. She talked about her income-generating activities and her participation in a women's organization that coordinated fertilizer and equipment purchases for the women's individual gardens. She supplemented her farming activities with gardening and by selling Ghanaian bread and watermelons. She was the only woman in Keru I had seen wearing jeans and makeup. Her husband left for Conakry,

Guinea, four years prior to our interview, while she continued to live in the village with their youngest son, who was six years old. She had given birth to four children, two of whom had died, one during childbirth and the other as a six-year-old from burns after his trousers caught fire. The oldest daughter had left the compound to marry, and the son, who suffered from anemia like Claire's child, regularly needed blood transfusions. Every time her son needed treatment, she had to take him to the hospital in town, about twenty-five kilometers from the village. She needed money for transport and for treatment, and she could not work in the fields when she was at the hospital. When she was unable to pay for the expenses herself, she asked her brothers for help.

Although Mouna was in regular contact with her husband, she knew almost nothing about his life in Guinea. She did not know if he was working or what kind of work he had. She did not know whether he had another wife in Guinea, and she did not know anything about his plans for the future. If she tried to call him, he did not answer the phone: "You are only able to hear news when a person answers the phone. If I call him, he does not answer." She continued: "I don't know what he is doing. He has told me nothing. I haven't asked him either. If you ask such questions, you risk discussing. This is how we are, the villagers; there is not transparency." Mouna's husband does not send money home on a regular basis. He only sent her money once, so that she could buy herself a bicycle. Mouna articulated herself well, and her answers to me were direct. It was clear that she was frustrated about her situation, having to manage by herself without financial support from her husband.

In 2017, I interviewed Abibou outside her in-laws' compound, where she lived. Abibou was in a special situation as she had not heard from her husband since he left the village to look for work in Guinea more than ten years earlier. At the time he left, their fourth child, a boy now twelve years old, had just learned to walk. Abibou had been farming the fields of her husband during his absence, and recently, because her husband had not been back for more than ten years, the village elders recognized her as the formal owner of the farmland.[10] It is very unusual for women to obtain land rights, but Abibou was supported by her father-in-law, who was angry with his son for not reporting back to the family. Abibou had been waiting for her husband all these years and was still waiting. Every time other migrants returned from Guinea, she asked them whether they had any news about her husband, but so far she had not had any success. The family members had not reported him missing to the police, Abibou said: "We implore God that he is still alive. I continue to look for him." She lived with her in-laws, who also supported her financially, particularly with expenses related to the schooling of her children. When I asked her how she managed, she replied: "It is simply a life of suffering." Abibou told me that she had a younger co-wife, but the co-wife had decided to leave the in-laws' household in order to remarry. When I asked Abibou whether she also considered remarrying, she replied: "There is nobody in the family with whom I could leave the children. I will stay and take care of my children." Thus, she had to stay and do the best she could to farm the land and hope for her husband's return.

The story of Abibou is (hopefully) not typical, but it is clear from my interviews that male mobility places the women staying behind in fragile positions facing uncertainties related to the unknown whereabouts of their husbands. As Boserup points out, extensive migration affects everyday life in rural villages in gendered ways. Women who stay behind are in a precarious situation as they engage in care labor, shoulder responsibility for children, and depend economically on other family members, including their in-laws, with whom they often live. They are left in a temporal and physical limbo. Despite the constraints on their mobility, they have to make many decisions about their household economy, the fields, their children's many illnesses, and the schooling of their children. They also have to decide whether to contact their husband, consult the dispensary, or start treatment of a sick child with home care. They are social actors with the capacity to act; some of them, like Mouna, make use of the sometimes-widened room for maneuver. But they act from a very fragile position, a position of structural vulnerability (Ribera and Hausmann-Muela 2011).

Absent-Present Husbands

When residents of Keru travel across national boundaries to seek work, the bonds to family members staying behind are not severed. Even though many male family members stay away for years, their role as absent-present husbands in their community of origin remains strong. They search for work in other countries—or in the main cities of Burkina—because, as Laurentine pointed out, "There is no work to find here." Many hopes and dreams are invested in the *aventure*, both for those leaving the community and for those staying behind. They all invest in the future through care labor. I have argued that Michel's journey to Libya was based on a desire to get away from the village for a while and a wish to succeed economically in order to return home, get married, and support his family. Likewise, Claire, Mouna, Abibou, and the many other wives who remained in the village during their husbands' absence worked hard to care for their children and tend the fields of their husbands. Many of the men who did not embark on *aventure* were to some extent also absent-present, as they moved between the provincial towns and the village in order to find temporary work or to do small-scale business. Because the remittances sent home were unpredictable, both in amount and timing, many wives engaged in other income-generating activities. Mouna sold bread and watermelons to cover food and health care expenses, and many other women grew tomatoes to sell directly at the local market or to Togolese merchants who had brought their own wares to sell at the Keru market.

Extensive migration affects everyday life in rural villages like Keru in very gendered ways. The stakes were high for the men leaving the village to find work in distant locations, as the case of Michel illustrates. Their journeys involved a number of uncertainties, including whether they would be able to find a job or secure an income that allowed them to send money home and start the construction of a new house. They might face long periods of hard work or long periods without work or with only occasional work. Some of them, like Michel, faced problems with their identity or employment documentation. Would they be harassed by the police, as happened to Laurentine, or by others during the high-risk journeys through weak states and through the Sahara Desert? Likewise, the women staying behind with the children lived extraordinarily tough lives with what I call *triple uncertainties*. Some of the migrants succeeded in saving money, constructing new houses, supporting the education of their children, and providing their wives with opportunities to develop their own businesses. However, most only managed to save a little, and an unknown number of others returned from their *aventures* without any savings at all.

Conclusion

As this chapter demonstrates, migration is part of everyday life in Keru. The Ebola epidemic, which closed the borders between various countries in the region, made Michel change plans. Instead of embarking on a journey to Guinea, Gabon, or Côte d'Ivoire, he and his family decided that he should travel north. Again in 2020, borders in the region were closed or restricted during the COVID-19 pandemic; this included Burkina Faso, where borders were closed for about four months as part of the country's epidemic control strategy.

Increasing pressure on land, high unemployment rates, and a weak state that does not provide social security benefits force many young people to go on high-risk *aventures*. The migrants' pathways and the duration of their stays are shaped by local, international, and global factors. The fact that Michel went to Libya and stayed for many years was triggered as much by external factors as by his own wishes. For Michel, as for many other men (and women), migrating is a way of mitigating their own and their families' fragile futures at home. However, the lives of the majority of the migrants and their families staying behind are precarious and full of uncertainties. Fathers who remain in the village are also often "absent-present" in relation to the everyday care labor. Although they may not travel far for employment, male household members are very mobile and often search for small-scale business activities outside of the village. Although some migrants succeed, the future looks fragile for those families whose members do not succeed with their *aventure*.

Notes

1. In *The Human Condition* (Arendt 2013), Arendt provides a complex, historical analysis of the three fundamental aspects of human life: labor, work, and action. She develops her analysis on the basis of ancient Greek philosophy in a discussion and critique of Karl Marx's analysis of human labor. Here, I draw only on Arendt's distinction between labor and work, as this distinction highlights the complex relationship between human activity as production (work) and a range of other activities, including reproduction and relational care.
2. UNICEF, "Migration Profiles: Burkina Faso." Retrieved 15 July 2023 from https://esa.un.org/miggmgprofiles/indicators/files/BurkinaFaso.pdf.
3. Unfortunately, we do not have data on the gender distribution of migrants from Keru. However, my observations confirm that the majority of people

migrating to Côte d'Ivoire and other West African countries from Keru are young men. In some cases, wives and children follow after the men have established themselves in the destination country, but in most cases, the wives stay in the village.

4. "I et hvilket som helst møde mellem mennesker ligger en uudtalt fordring, uanset under hvilke omstændigheder mødet finder sted og hvilken karakter det har." My translation.
5. International Organization for Migration (UN), "IOM Helps Stranded Burkina Faso Migrants to Return Home from Libya," 23 September 2016. Retrieved 15 July 2023 from https://www.iom.int/news/iom-helps-stranded-burkina-faso-migrants-return-home-libya.
6. The kola nut plays an important symbolic role in this region. It is used as a gift to show hospitality, friendship, and respect. When visiting elderly people or the chief in Keru, I often brought a number of kola nuts to show my respect.
7. I am aware that the term "left behind" may suggest that those who remain in the village have little agency. I try to use the terms "remain" or "stay behind" instead, as my analysis shows that they take upon themselves a huge responsibility and show a lot of agency.
8. This section is based primarily on a series of interviews with women "staying behind" in Keru. In addition to a number of informal conversations with women in the village, I conducted fourteen in-depth interviews with women whose husbands were working outside of Burkina Faso.
9. Bread is not part of everyday meals in Keru; however, many people like bread from Ghana because of its soft texture and sweet taste.
10. In rural Burkina Faso, land is not private property, but land rights are inherited from father to sons. User rights to land are distributed through inheritance, and land disputes are usually solved by the chief and the elders in the village. Serious land disputes may also be taken to court.

Part II

Technologies of Care

Chapter 4
Technologies and Cosmologies

La Vaccinatrice

I first met Mariam Salemporgo in 1996 during my first long-term stay in the village of Keru. She lived with her husband and son, along with her co-wife and children, in a small compound close to the marketplace and to Thomas's household. Mariam was called *la vaccinatrice*, as she specialized in the prevention and treatment of children's stomach problems by rubbing herbal medicines into incisions that she made. Mariam did not provide her services publicly at the market like many other local herbalists, but instead "vaccinated" children every Monday morning in her courtyard. Mariam was an elderly, physically solid woman, with a brightly colored scarf always covering her hair. She was quite social and often attended Beatrice's millet beer *cabaret*. Mariam and her family cultivated their small plots of land like most other citizens in the village. Farming in this region of Africa is hard work and economically precarious, so most families also own a few cattle, goats, or pigs and a number of chickens to help make ends meet, but remittances from migrant work are becoming a more and more important supplement for many families. Mariam and her family lived mainly from subsistence farming complemented by income from her son's temporary jobs in a nearby town. Mariam belonged to the minority Catholic community in the village and often wore a cotton dress with printed Christian symbols and a cross on a leather string around her neck. When visiting Keru, I often passed by her compound to say hello—she appreciated the attention and was always very welcoming.

When I arrived at Mariam's compound one Monday morning in 1997 before 7:00 a.m., a small group was already waiting under the shelter outside her compound. Many patients came from distant villages and had been up very early in order to make it to Mariam's compound. I found Mariam inside the courtyard, busy preparing the herbal medicines for the day's treatments. She kneeled on the ground, pounding burned herbs into a black powder in a calabash. She used bark from a number of different trees and bushes that she collected herself in the bush outside the village. During one of our conversations, she mentioned the names of five specific trees she took bark from, and I managed to identify them in the book *Trees and Plants of the Sahel* (von Maydell 1986). A day or two before the consultations, she burned the bark into charcoal, then every Monday morning before starting the consultations she pounded the charcoal on a broken piece of calabash until it became a fine-grained powder. Before she started to vaccinate, she usually put on a T-shirt and a clean *pagne*.

This Monday morning, the first patient was a small boy two or three years old. The boy's stomach was swollen, and the mother was keen to get him treated. He looked malnourished, with thin arms and legs and a ballooned stomach. While the child sat on his mother's lap, Mariam took half a razor blade and quickly made a number of small cuts on the skin of the child's stomach. The cuts began to bleed, the blood soon running down the boy's stomach, and he cried intensely. The mother comforted her son, talking softly to him while Mariam took some of the black medical powder and smeared it onto the boy's stomach, mixing it with the blood. I found it unpleasant to observe this treatment—hearing the boy's cries and seeing Mariam mix the powder with the blood on the boy's stomach—though she performed the treatment with professionalism, and it only took four or five minutes. Immediately after the treatment, a piece of cloth was bandaged around the boy's stomach and he was put to the breast of his mother, who looked relieved as he was quickly soothed. Mariam gave us a big smile, probably sensing the tense atmosphere, then instructed the young mother to come back for two more rounds of "vaccination" in order for it to be effective. She then invited the next patient into the courtyard. According to Mariam, some children carry a stomach disease from birth, having acquired it when their pregnant mother carelessly ate mangos or other sweet fruits. When this happens, the child is born with the mother's stomach problems. Therefore, pregnant women should avoid eating sweet fruits, Mariam noted.

The last patient this morning was a small two-month-old girl, who was to be vaccinated against *Liula*, a well-known and feared disease in the region. The girl was naked except for a small pair of panties and was held by her mother, who seemed eager for her daughter to be treated. Mariam performed the vaccination quickly, making many small cuts on the child's stomach and back with the razor blade. Like the previous patient, the child cried loudly but stopped almost immediately when she started breastfeeding. The mother looked very relieved and happy sitting with her daughter on her lap after this rather dramatic treatment. Mariam carefully explained that the vaccinated child would get diarrhea and in that way expel the disease. The disease, called *Niula/Liula* (literally meaning "bird"), is understood by people in the area to be quite dangerous. The sick child gets strong convulsions that resemble birds flapping their wings and is explained by many villagers to be caused by a bird flying above a child or pregnant woman as they sleep outdoors at night. The practice of vaccinating against the disease was widespread in the region (Charmillot 1997).

I worried about the hygiene during the intervention, particularly when Mariam used the razor blade; I was unsure whether the same blade was reused for more than one treatment. However, Mariam assured me that everything was under control. None of her patients had returned after a failed treatment. She was confident that the skill of treating specific diseases was a special gift, a "richness" passed on from her grandmother. "It is my treasure," she explained. Mariam did not, however, earn a lot as *vaccinatrice*. The parents of the vaccinated children paid 165 CFA [franc] and a rooster for treating a boy and 220 CFA [franc] (around US$0.50) and a hen for a girl. The payments for girls and boys were different, reflecting the numbers four and three (girls needed four treatments, while boys needed three).[1]

In this chapter, I begin by exploring similarities and differences between the local incision technique practiced by Mariam Salemporgo in the village of Keru and the vaccination services provided by the rural dispensary. I discuss the role of various techniques and technologies used on the body to protect and strengthen it, including the widespread use of amulets among both Muslims and Christians. My aim here is not to compare the biomedical approach with traditional systems of thought, as many earlier medical anthropological studies of health care in Africa have (Evans-Pritchard 1937; Feierman and Janzen 1992; Finkler 1994; Janzen 1978). Instead, I focus on care practices in a broader context where various preventive and therapeutic technologies are used to nurse relationships between the individual and society. I argue that these technologies involve tending relations with the state in order to secure access to public health services and cultivating relations with non-human agents in order to confirm connections to the spiritual world.

Mothers invest time and money in these social relationships and even consult specialists when their children are healthy. From their perspective, both types of vaccination are prevenient practices that protect against future diseases and strengthen connections with the staff at the dispensary as well as with the spirits. The relationship to the nurses at the dispensary is often fragile. Mothers often fear being blamed for arriving too late for consultation.[2] Likewise, it is notoriously difficult to know how to avoid the malevolent action of spirits. Thus, by getting their children vaccinated at the dispensary and at the local *vaccinatrice*, mothers both *care for* their children and *care about* the social relations with agents who possess power that may affect the future health of their children. Through these preventive and therapeutic practices, the people of Keru endorse their belonging to the state as well as to the local cosmology.

Preventive Incision Techniques

Mariam's expertise included treatment of diseases, such as headaches and stomach problems, and preventive vaccination, as in the case of *Liula*. On another Monday morning when I was visiting, a mother had come to get her two- or three-month-old baby vaccinated. Mariam used the same incision technique as she had before, making small cuts with a razor blade on the child's stomach. In this case, she also made cuts on the forehead, the chest, the lower back, the wrists, and the top of the child's feet. The child cried while Mariam was doing the cutting, and the mother held him firmly, soothing him. Mariam again quickly smeared a black powder made of ashes from herbs into the many small wounds, ensuring that it was mixed with the blood. After the treatment, a piece of cloth was put around the child, and he was allowed to breastfeed. Mariam was confident that the child would be fine. Although Mariam and most of the other local healers I met did not want to share the "secrets" of their specific healing qualifications, they welcomed my interest in their knowledge and practice. My long-term acquaintance with Thomas and Jean probably also helped, and many of the residents in Keru knew me and were well aware of my interest in village life and local health care practices. I was, in a sense, recognized as outside of the local medical field.

On another occasion, I observed a pair of siblings being vaccinated. The girl was about eight years old, the boy ten. They were both very nervous; the girl started crying before Mariam even began cutting. As this girl had already gotten one of her four rounds of treatment, she was quite aware of what was going to happen. While Mariam performed her treatment, the girl was held firmly by Jean, who knew Mariam and the other local healers very well. In addition to smearing the medicines on the girl's bleeding stomach, Mariam also gave the girl a small amount of the powder orally four times. Having observed the treatment of his sister, the boy started to cry, but Mariam resolutely continued. She finalized the treatment by giving him a little medicine orally three times, as three is the number for males. These two children did not have swollen stomachs, and they were not sick. They were both vaccinated preventively against a disease called *Lougouré*, literally meaning "the side of the stomach," which a child might be born with or might acquire if not purged regularly or if breastfed before defecating after an enema. Mariam explained that it is important to defecate before breastfeeding in order to prevent the enema water from causing sickness. I happened to meet the vaccinated girl about five years later. She showed me the very small scars on her stomach and assured me that she had never suffered from *Lougouré*.

Mariam was one of many local herbalists in the village treating stomach problems and fevers. However, she was quite unique, and well known in the area, for her preventive incisions. Mariam continued her vaccination and treatment practices every Monday morning for many, many years, treating between four and ten children every week, some from very far away. Mariam passed away in 2016 at the age of almost eighty after having suffered a stroke. She was hospitalized at the local dispensary for a week with one side of her body paralyzed before passing away. However, as in the case of many other local healers, she managed to transfer her skills to her daughter, who took up the routine Monday morning vaccination practices in Keru.

Vaccination Policy in Burkina Faso

Burkina Faso was the first African country to use the measles vaccine, starting with a mass vaccination campaign in 1962. Vaccinations against measles continued during the 1960s, mainly during mass campaigns, although the coverage remained relatively low. The Expanded Program of Immunization (EPI) was launched worldwide in 1974 with the overall aim of making immunization against diphtheria, pertussis, tetanus, poliomyelitis, measles, and tuberculosis available to every child in the world by 1990 (Keja et al. 1988). Worldwide, the immunization program has been a success: smallpox is eradicated, polio cases have decreased by 99 percent since 1988 (Venkatesan 2022),[3] and about 85 percent of children globally have received all three doses of the DPT (diphtheria, tetanus, pertussis) vaccine.[4] It is considered to be the most successful public health care intervention ever in terms of the number of deaths prevented (Kagoné et al. 2017). According to the official 2018 estimate, in Burkina Faso around 91 percent of children under twelve months old have received the third dose of the DPT vaccine.[5]

While mass immunization programs do not have a long history in Africa, the practice of vaccinating against specific diseases does. Variolations against smallpox were practiced in West Africa long before being introduced in Europe. Variolation (also known as inoculation) is a technique of infecting a patient with fluids from a smallpox pustule, thus making the person immune to smallpox (Stewart and Devlin 2006). In 1716, Cotton Mather wrote the earliest known report on variolation in West Africa based on information provided to him by an African he had enslaved (Imperato 1977; Riedel 2005), and Mather later introduced the technique in the American colonies. Mungo Park, an explorer who traveled along the Niger River in the eighteenth century, recorded the existence of variolations in the Gambia (Imperato 1977; Samuelsen 2001). In Africa, variolation was only practiced during smallpox outbreaks and was not performed in routine vaccination campaigns.

The EPI was introduced to Burkina Faso in 1980–81, and in 1983–84, the new revolutionary government under Thomas Sankara launched the "Vaccination Commando" mass campaign in collaboration with UNICEF. The campaign became part of the revolutionary rhetoric, emphasizing that immunization protects the family and should be seen as part of a mother's caretaking duties toward her children. Vaccinations were also seen as an important contribution to building a strong country, making children "as strong as a commando." The campaign was intense: village and district committees were organized with the responsibility of preparing lists of children to be vaccinated; guides for health workers, schoolteachers, and parents were distributed; posters and flyers were widely circulated; and radio campaigns were organized to communicate the campaign to all corners of the country (UNICEF 1985). The campaign was organized through the Committees for the Defense of the Revolution (CDRs), which had replaced the previous political structure at all levels of the country. During a three-week period in 1984, about 730,000 children aged nine months to six years were vaccinated against measles, and approximately 1.7 million children aged one to fourteen were vaccinated against yellow fever and meningitis (Kessler et al. 1986). It was a huge and impressive intervention in a poor country with an otherwise weak infrastructure. Vaccination programs were also prioritized during the twenty-seven years of Blaise Compaoré's governance with continued strong support from UNICEF and GAVI (now known as Gavi, the Vaccine Alliance). Today, immunization is part of the primary health care program with vaccination services based at the dispensaries, known as Centres de Santé et de Promotion Sociale (CSPS), where vaccination days are organized regularly, with catch-up days for those who missed the regular sessions. UNICEF and Gavi provide the vaccines free of charge (Kagoné et al. 2017).

Vaccinations at the Dispensary

Since the 1980s, nurses based at the peripheral health dispensaries have administered vaccination programs. While the general utilization of government health services in Burkina Faso is relatively low,[6] there is an active demand for vaccinations among rural citizens, especially mothers, and vaccination rates are high. Since the introduction of mass vaccination campaigns in low- and middle-income countries in the mid-1970s, the government of Burkina Faso has prioritized the development and implementation of a national immunization program following international guidelines.

The coverage rate in Burkina Faso has increased significantly over the years. A study by Moubassira Kagoné and colleagues published in 2017 showed that 80 percent of all children are fully vaccinated at the age of twelve months.[7] Interestingly, the coverage rate was found to be higher in rural areas than in urban settlements (Kagoné et al. 2017). Nobila Ouédraogo, Moubassira Kagoné, Ali Sié, Heiko Becher, and Olaf Müller (2013) also found high vaccination coverage in a study using the existing Health and Demographic Surveillance System to assess vaccination rates among 11,906 children under five years old in Nouna health district. Here, it was estimated that 81 percent of children aged twelve to twenty-three months were fully immunized, and 91 percent of children under five years old had received at least one vaccination. Roughly two-thirds of the households could show a vaccination card: about 85 percent of families with infants and 45 percent of families with children four to five years old (N. Ouédraogo et al. 2013). Burkina Faso follows the WHO preventable vaccine program and has added a number of vaccines to its routine vaccination program, most recently the meningococcal A vaccine, which was added in 2017. This new vaccine will hopefully contribute to a reduction of meningitis cases, as outbreaks of meningitis have been a huge problem in Burkina Faso as well as in some of the other countries in the Central Sahel, with severe epidemics every two to three years. Most vaccines are given at eight, twelve, and sixteen weeks of age, followed by other vaccines at nine and fifteen months. Thus, the ordinary vaccination program includes a total of five visits to the dispensary within the first fifteen months of life, which is quite a demanding schedule, particularly when considering that these five visits are supposed to be carried out at times when the child is not sick.

The routine vaccination days at the rural dispensaries serve not only as important health interventions but also as important social events. Women leave their households very early in the morning, forming long queues outside the dispensaries hours before the nurses begin working. I often observed the narrow benches outside the clinics in Tenga and Keru occupied by waiting mothers and children. The mothers, who were dressed up, often took the opportunity to chat with women from their own village or from neighboring villages as they waited. The women showed up early in the hopes that they would be able to get the vaccinations quickly, not spending too much time at the health facility, and then return home early in order to continue their other daily tasks. On vaccination days, the dispensary buzzed with activities, mothers coming and going, children crying after the vaccination prick, and health staff deeply engaged in their work. The catchment area of a rural dispensary in Burkina Faso includes up to twelve villages, which means that many women walk a long distance. The two nurses at the dispensary are busy on vaccination days: one is usually fully occupied with vaccinations while the other takes care of the other patients. When the supply of motorcycles and gasoline is stable, the nurses provide outreach vaccination services to those villages in their catchment area that are located far from the dispensary.

Vaccination Card: Signature of the Absent-Present State

The completed vaccinations are noted on the child's vaccination card, a very important document given to the mother at her first antenatal care visit. The card is used to note basic information about the mother at the antenatal visits as well as information about the child, including birth weight (if known) and vaccinations. It is a kind of state "signature" recognizing citizenship (a status of belonging) and stipulating the expectations to be fulfilled as a good client or patient of the public health care system (such as attending the next vaccination session) (Das and Poole 2004: 225–251; Street 2012).

Inspired by Jacques Derrida, Das emphasizes that writing is more than an extension of oral communication. Writing is a way of communicating with absent persons but also has the potential to introduce a gap between a rule and its performance. The vaccination card and other documents, such as the identity card, show "how the state comes [to] be present in the everyday life of its subjects. . . . It is precisely because the documents can be forged and used out of context, and because the bureaucratic-legal processes are not legible even to those responsible for implementing them that the state can penetrate the life of the community and yet remain elusive" (Das and Poole 2004: 245). The notion of *signature* is particularly relevant in this context, as it helps us understand the complex relationship between the state and its citizens. As mentioned earlier, the state is, as seen from a rural citizen's perspective, both absent and present. It is absent in the sense that the few governmental institutions located in rural areas are almost empty, and often the staff is absent.

At the same time, it is present through representations such as the vaccination and identity cards, which clearly symbolize a relationship between the individual citizen and the state.[8] The vaccination card bears state rules and procedures and materializes a "spectral" presence of the state.

The rural citizens are quite aware of the importance of such documents. To the individual mother, the vaccination card is precious, and it is usually stored in a safe place within the household. However, in the rural areas of Burkina Faso where many people are illiterate, this "signature" of the state also communicates an alienation or estrangement of the citizens from the state. The rural mothers know that this is an important document, but many of them are not able to read or understand the text noted on the cards. The vaccination card not only represents the state as a rational-bureaucratic organization but also provides the state with a magical presence in the community. Moreover, it exposes the vulnerability and fragile positions of the rural citizens. Losing the card, or not protecting it well, may give the mother troubles at the next visit to the dispensary, including the risk of being scolded by the nurse.

Vaccination as a Medical Technology

As mentioned at the beginning of this chapter, the basic conceptual and explanatory frameworks of the two types of vaccination—the government-led vaccination program and Mariam's vaccination practices—are very different. One is based on a biomedical conception of infusing small doses of antigens into an otherwise healthy body to mobilize resistance toward a specific disease, while the other is based on an indigenous practice of infusing local herbal medicine into the body in order to stop a potential, perhaps inborn disease from emerging. However, there are also a number of similarities. Both "services" are routinized, they operate professionally with fixed vaccination days, and patients must wait in line for their appointments. There is also resemblance between the two incision techniques: in both cases, the skin is penetrated by sharp instruments, whether needles or razor blades, that are manufactured and imported. Both techniques infuse a medical substance that is mixed with bodily fluids. The local incision technique, in which a substance is rubbed into the body, is based on an old practice in Burkina Faso, while the biomedical vaccination technique is relatively new. The resonance between the two incision practices corresponds with local understandings of bodily processes and good childcare. Furthermore, vaccination as a preventive measure, where children's healthy bodies are worked upon in order to promote health, corresponds with other local practices, such as regularly giving small children enemas, as described in chapter 2.

The two vaccination practices may even have influenced one another. The "Vaccination Commando" campaign in the early 1980s instantiated a direct relationship between being a good revolutionary citizen, a "vaccination commando," and having one's children vaccinated. Several studies have documented the dynamic relationship between technologies and innovations introduced from outside and certain indigenous practices. This has been shown in relation to medical technologies, such as injections and medicines (Van der Geest and Whyte 1988; Van der Geest, Whyte, and Hardon 1996; Whyte, Van der Geest, and Hardon 2002), as well as social technologies, such as confession, as described very eloquently by Vinh-Kim Nguyen in his analysis of community organizations' responses to the HIV epidemic (Nguyen 2010). Another important similarity is that both practices concoct a "signature." The "signature of the state" in the routine vaccination practices at the public health facility takes the form of the vaccination card (with only small marks, if any, on the body), while the scars resulting from the vaccination practices of *la vaccinatrice* become a "signature" of the local cosmology inscribed on the skin. Mariam's qualifications are based not only on her technical skills and knowledge about how and where to make the small cuts and how to prepare the medicines, but also on her "magical" skills and knowledge about the spiritual world.

Cicatrization or scarification[9] with knifes or razors has been reported in many classical anthropological field studies in Africa (Buckley 1985; Imperato 1977; Janzen 1978; V. Turner 1967). Variolations were often referred to in local languages as "indigenous vaccinations" (Imperato 1977: 170). Many of the elderly people in Keru, including Thomas and Beatrice, have clearly marked facial scars. The particular scarification patterns are often said to reflect clan or ethnic affiliation—in their case, affiliation with the Bissa. In his analysis of Tiv markings, Paul Bohannan claimed that they conferred membership in a social group (quoted in Rubin 1988). I am not sure if the explanation is that simple; the markings might also reflect former aesthetic ideals or may have originated from social categories used during the colonial past. In any case, inscriptions on the body, like these scars, are open for interpretation. There may be no simple reading of the skin, as Megan Vaughan emphasizes, but the scars "mark the relationship between the individual and society, between the present and the past, between living persons and their ancestors, between the rulers and the ruled" (Vaughan 2007: 386). The current vaccination routines, both those authorized by the state and those that are part of tradition, express relationships between the individual and society.[10]

Amulets and Other Technologies

Many children in Keru wear amulets around the neck or waist. The amulets usually consist of a small leather "package" with a medical substance or an inscription from the Qur'an written on a small piece of paper inside. According to Robert Handloff, amulets might also include a *katemi*, a quadrangle divided into smaller squares, each of which contains a number, a word, or a letter with a numerical value (Handloff 1982). The amulets are often produced by local marabouts (Qur'anic specialists), who treat patients and produce these preventive devices. Like the enemas and the vaccinations, amulets serve to protect children from future malaise. During a series of interviews with mothers of sick children in 2001, one mother told us that she had lost six of her children to illness, with only two children left alive. She had now provided the youngest child with a protective amulet and, when the child had a swollen stomach, administered enemas with water. The mother furthermore explained that when the child felt sick from *yingwingre* (warm body), she usually consulted Dr. Sorgho,[11] a retired nurse in a neighboring village, who would provide the child with a series of injections. For this mother, as for most of the other women in Keru I have talked with, it is not a question of selecting between so-called traditional medicine or biomedicine. Mothers consider each case of sickness carefully and decide how best to take care of the child. Decisions are often pragmatic, depending on previous experiences, availability of cash for potential payments at the health facility, knowledge about relevant herbal plants, and individual assessments of specific symptoms.

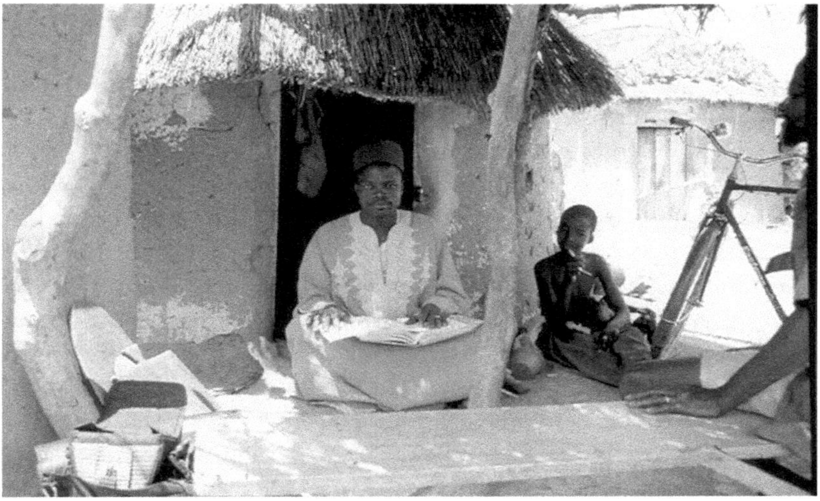

Figure 4.1. Marabout in front of his house, Burkina Faso (© Helle Samuelsen 2023)

The amulets often serve as general protection, though I also encountered a few marabouts who made amulets to protect against specific diseases, such as whooping cough and measles. One of them explained carefully how he wrote specific quotes from the Qur'an on a leaf from the Kuilenga tree. When writing the quotations, he placed the leaf on a small piece of wood from the same type of tree. After writing on the leaf, he folded it carefully and fastened it with a thin thread before it was sewn into a small piece of leather. Before touching the Qur'an, he washed his face, hands, and feet. He explained that the amulet "is actually a kind of vaccination." Both measles and whooping cough are transmitted by saliva, he said, so a child might transmit the disease to another child if drinking from the same calabash. Although his own children had only been vaccinated by him and not at the dispensary, he did not see the two vaccination practices as antagonistic.

Another very old—and locally famous—traditional healer explained that he also used quotations from the Qur'an as a therapeutic technology. These quotations were not parceled into amulets, but washed into water that was used to treat the patient. This man, who lived outside Tenga, claimed to be more than one hundred years old when I first met him in 1997. Dressed in a long brown garment that covered his thin legs and feet, he indeed looked very old as he sat cross-legged in the shade on a plastic mat outside his small house. He spoke slowly, but he mumbled and was quite hard to understand, as he had few remaining teeth. He was one of the few specialists I met who claimed to treat mental illnesses. He would start his treatment by selecting specific verses from the Qur'an, which he then wrote down on a small wooden board with a thin stick dipped in ink. Then, he selected pieces of bark from five different kinds of trees and soaked the pieces in water. The wooden board with the verses was then washed with the bark-infused water, and the letters "fell" down into the water. The mentally ill patient was then told to drink some of the herbal water and wash with it. This treatment would cure the patient, the marabout claimed. Over the years, he told me, he has treated many sick people, perhaps fifteen to twenty people a year. People came all the way from Ouagadougou and other provinces. The same technology of washing verses from the Qur'an into an herbal liquid to treat mentally ill patients was explained by another marabout, who added musk and camphor, along with herbs, to the liquid. *Zin*, spirits living on small hills or near rocks, may inflict mental illness on those walking in the bush, he explained. It is a common belief in this area that such spirits must be treated with respect, as they may inflict mental illness or other harm on those who happen to meet or bump into them or insult them in some other way. Among the many traditional healers I encountered, only marabouts claimed to be able to treat mental illness; others tended to focus on other specific diseases or symptoms.

Tending Non-Human Relations

In Arnold van Gennep's definition of rites of passage, the thresholds between spaces are crucial: "Whoever passes [the threshold] from one [zone] to the other finds himself physically and magico-religiously in a special situation for a certain length of time: he wavers between two worlds" (Van Gennep 2013: 19). Transitions are significant for local interpretations of sickness and for local therapeutic practices among the Bissa. Sickness itself is a transition in which the sick person wavers between two worlds. Scholars have pointed to a perceptual distinction between domestic space and bush space in West African societies (Cartry 1979; Fainzang 1986;

Gottlieb 2012; Van Beek and Banga 2002). As described elsewhere (Samuelsen 1999), the borders and boundaries between village and bush are fluid. Each is a "practiced place," to use Michel de Certeau's distinction between space and place (1988: 117), and the boundaries between the two change according to the practices taking place. According to the marabouts around Keru and Tenga, there are both good and bad *zin* spirits. The good spirits help the marabouts in their healing practices, while the bad spirits may cause harm—usually mental illness—if disturbed. The *zin* spirits live in the bush and, though generally not visible, are usually described as tall and white. According to Sylvie Fainzang, *zin* (or, in Bissa, *zina*) have been integrated into the Bissa cosmology through the growing number of Muslims in the region (Fainzang 1986).[12]

The following is a short passage from an interview with an indigenous herbalist, Abdoul, where we talk about the *zin* spirits:

> *Helle*: I have heard that there exist sprits who are capable of provoking illness. Could you explain this?
>
> *Abdoul*: Yes, there are actually spirits who provoke certain illnesses.
>
> *Helle*: How does this happen?
>
> *Abdoul*: When someone arrives home after having met a spirit, that person will start to tremble and behave like a fool. In that case, it is important to start treatment as soon as possible.
>
> *Helle*: Where do you meet the spirits?
>
> *Abdoul*: The spirits like open spaces. If a person likes going those places, she may meet them. One can also meet them during a walk. It is during these encounters that they bring about sickness.
>
> *Helle*: But it is not possible to see the spirits?
>
> *Abdoul*: No, one cannot see them.
>
> *Helle*: How are the spirits? Do they look like human beings or like animals?
>
> *Abdoul*: They look like human beings. They are dressed in white.
>
> *Helle*: Have you seen a spirit?
>
> *Abdoul*: If it is not during the night, it is not possible to see them.
>
> *Helle*: But at night then, is it possible to see them?
>
> *Abdoul*: If your path crosses their path during night, you see them; they disappear immediately.

Helle: Are they also able to "attack" you during daytime?

Abdoul: During the day with full sunlight, you cannot see them, but they see us. At that moment, they might cause illness.

Helle: At noon?

Abdoul: Yes, at noon or during nighttime.

Helle: Why do the spirits attack human beings? Because one has done something wrong, or what?

Abdoul: There are two types of spirits, one kind of spirit cause misfortune and they are evil. If you meet a bad one, even if you have not done anything wrong, it will bring sickness, *a yôkda foo* [literally, in Mooré, "it attacks you"]. When you meet the spirits, if they want to bring sickness, you will know. Immediately, your body will freeze, and you will start trembling.

As the extract illustrates, the spirits of the bush are quite powerful and dangerous. Trees are another non-human agent that may cause sickness. Sickness caused by tree spirits, which might enter human space at night, is referred to as *tiisi* (Mooré) or *go* (Bissa), both of which literally mean "tree." Illnesses called *tiisi* are not characterized by one specific symptom but share features such as skin changes and swelling. Sometimes, when related to an illness of the skin, *tiisi* is translated locally as *gale* (scabies). A marabout explained that if a woman dreams that she's making love to her husband, she's really making love to a spirit, which will instigate irregular and very painful menses during which her blood will be black. If a man has such a dream, he will start feeling pain when urinating (Samuelsen 2004a). A disease called *waofo* (snake in Mooré) in which the skin looks like snakeskin is also caused by a spirit. A child might get this disease if a pregnant woman happens to cross the track of a python. It is not the snake itself that transmits the disease but a spirit in the form of a snake.

Although both Islam and Christianity have many devotees in this area (with a majority of Muslims), everyday life in the villages also includes many practices and interpretations of sicknesses that relate to non-human agents. Women who have twins perform a sacrifice to the spirits once a year in order to maintain good relations with the *kinkirsi* (the twin spirits). The local diviner, whom I met at the beginning of my fieldwork, was almost blind and used to live outside the village in a small hut. He was famous in the local area for his divining skills and, during divination, stayed in close contact with the *kinkirsi*, the twin spirits. His grandfather, who could also communicate with the *kinkirsi*, had managed to install them in two small jars, which the diviner placed just next to the goatskin where he sat during the rite. The jars, turned upside down, were covered with chicken feathers, clotted blood, and other remains from previous sacrifices. When performing the divination, the diviner first called upon the spirits while shaking a calabash with seeds to get their attention. Following the divination, the person who sought advice was often asked to perform one or more sacrifices to the spirits. In my own case, the diviner asked me to buy a chicken and some eggs and sacrifice them at a spot where two paths crossed. After the death of this diviner, the villagers began to consult another diviner living in another village, quite far away from Keru.

The Craft of Bonesetting

Treating fractures was mainly seen as a craft that could be acquired through apprenticeship with a bonesetting practitioner. However, the bonesetters in this area also have a special relationship with the twin spirits, who play an important role in the local myth of bonesetting. Here is the story told by one of the bonesetters in Keru:

> This is the story of the bonesetters. Once upon a time there was a woman and her co-wife who lived with their husband. One day one of the women asked her co-wife for a calabash for her work. Unfortunately, the calabash broke. She told her co-wife and apologized. Then she took some thread and sewed the calabash with great care. The co-wife refused the calabash. Then the first co-wife went to buy a brand new calabash to replace the broken one. However, the wicked co-wife refused it, and said she would accept nothing but the original calabash, but with no cracks. "Give me back the calabash you borrowed from me, but without any breaks or deformations."
>
> The good lady went to seek advice from her husband, who could say nothing but advise her to fulfill the wish of the co-wife. Equipped with the broken calabash, the woman entered the bush in tears. After several days of walking and overcoming a number of obstacles, she encountered some spirits from the bush, who asked her what she was looking for so far from the village and why she was in tears. Trembling with fright, she told them about her misery. The spirits, the *kinkirsi*, gave her some medicine

> and told her to put it inside the calabash and then replace the broken piece. If she respected that, the spirits told her, the calabash would be repaired after seven days and no one would notice the break anymore. Back home, the woman followed the recommendations, and, after seven days, the calabash was healed. When the spirits gave her the products, they told her that if the calabash was repaired at the seventh day, she could use the same recommendations to heal any type of fracture.
>
> However, the patient must respect some prohibitions. He must refrain from eating meat, peanuts, pancakes, and beignets, and refrain from drinking *dolo* until he is completely healed. When healed, he must pay for the treatment, four chickens and a sum of 220 CFA [franc] if it concerns a woman and three chickens and 165 CFA [franc] if the patient is a male. At that time, we must also shave the head of the patient, which will then allow him to eat again all that was forbidden to him. On the day that his head is shaved, all the forbidden products must be prepared and poured on the fetishes in honor of the helping spirits. The sum of money should also be deposited on the fetishes.[13]

The medicines provided by the *kinkirsi* to the woman with the broken calabash in this myth are identical to the medicines used by the bonesetters in Keru to heal fractures. Zambédé, another bonesetter, explained his treatment in the following way:

> If the fracture is at the thigh, I first of all make an exact localization of the fracture. Then I ask another person to help me to pull the leg in order to reposition the fracture. When the thigh is back in a normal position, I start to massage it until all the bones are back in place. Then I immobilize the leg and bandage it. After two days, I check to see if the bones are back in the normal position. If all is well, I check it again after two days until the seventh day. At day eight, I boil some water—it has to be very hot—it should burn my fingers. I scrub the leg with Karité butter first with my hands, then with a piece of cloth. I have to be very careful that the hot water does not burn the thigh, as this could provoke another disease. I do this every third day until it is healed.

In most cases, he said, the fractures are caused by falling from a tree. If the person has lost a lot of blood, he refers the patient to the dispensary. When the patient returns, he continues the treatment of the fracture. Health professionals at the dispensaries and the district hospital generally recognize the skills of the bonesetters, praising their treatment. The knowledge of the bonesetters was usually passed from father to son; it was privileged knowledge that not

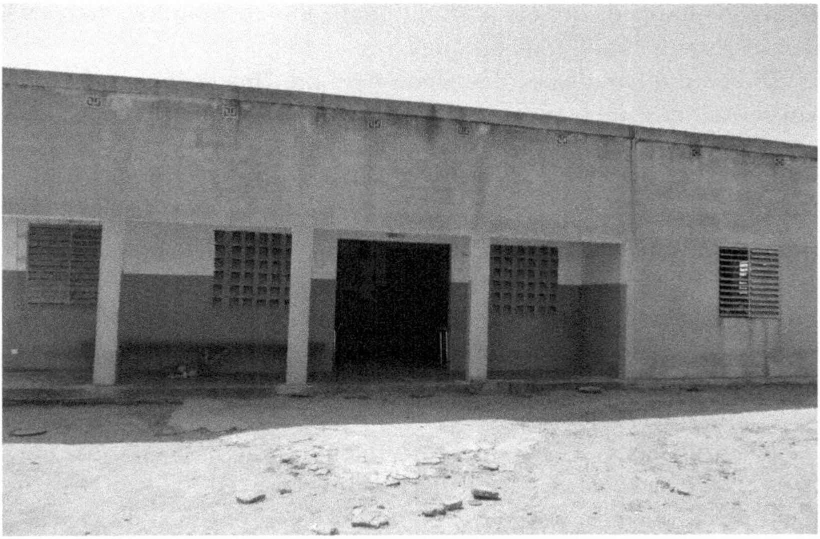

Figure 4.2. Rural dispensary, Burkina Faso (© Helle Samuelsen 2023)

everybody could be told about. There was also some secrecy around the various medical products used during treatment, as one of the bonesetters told me: "However, I am prohibited from revealing the secret to anyone without authorization. If I started to tell you what products I use, then one day, faced with a case of a fracture, you start treating it. That would have very negative consequences because you are not initiated and are not a bonesetter. Besides, if I showed you the products, the spirits would get angry with you and you would get fractures and then you would come to be treated here at my place."

Signatures of Belonging

In Keru and Tenga, mothers consult a diversity of practitioners, who use a number of techniques and technologies to prevent sickness and to care for sick children. In this chapter, I focused on two vaccination practices, the "local" vaccination practice performed by Mariam Salemporgo and the biomedical vaccination provided at the public health dispensary. In addition, I examined the use of amulets and the technologies of bonesetting and divination.[14] As noted at the beginning of the chapter, my aim here is not to compare systems of thought—biomedical versus traditional—but to examine the practice of various (bodily) techniques.

The care technologies described here are "magical" in a Maussian sense, inasmuch as "the effect derives from something else, and usually this is not of the same order" (Mauss 2001: 25). Marcel Mauss explains: "Thus, in medical practices, words, incantations, ritual and astrological observances are magical: this is the realm of the occult and of the sprits, a world of ideas which imbues ritual movements and gestures with a special kind of effectiveness" (2001: 25). In other words, it is not the marabout's technique of writing surahs from the Qur'an that by itself makes the ritual effective; there is something more to it. Likewise, it is not the technology of vaccination itself, whether done by the local *vaccinatrice* or in the dispensary, that makes it effective. In such practices there is more to the treatment rituals than the technique itself. The nurse, the local *vaccinatrice*, and the marabout all have special skills that are either acquired or inherited. Magical rites are carried out in secret; even when a magician has to work in public, he "makes an attempt to dissemble: his gestures become furtive and his words indistinct, 'spells' or 'prescriptions' are muttered in order to guard his power/his special gift" (Levi-Strauss 1963). This is the case in many of the so-called traditional healing rituals as well as in the practices at the public dispensary, where the nurse rarely explains the diagnosis or the prescription. The consultations take the form of a routinized ritual, where the magician, whether nurse, *vaccinatrice*, or marabout, both guard and demonstrate their power.

Vaccination technologies of all sorts are about penetrating the skin with the purpose of mixing medical substances with bodily fluids in order to prevent people from falling ill with specific diseases. In the case of public health vaccinations, they are also about responding to the demands of the state and tending social relationships with the state. These relationships are confirmed through the vaccination card, which serves as a kind of state signature. I encountered many women who were very anxious that they would be criticized by the nurse if their card had become crumpled or dirty. The mothers know how important this card is for obtaining future access to public health services. In the case of the local *vaccinatrice*, the relationship to non-human beings and the local cosmology is tended. The use of these different but comparable technologies marks relationships between the individual and society.

Likewise, other technologies, such as amulets, herbal liquid mixed with verses of the Qur'an, or other local therapies, also care for the relationship between the individual and non-human beings. As described above, many of these techniques work with the borders between human (domestic) space and non-human (bush) space.

Conclusion

Many studies of medical pluralism and therapeutic trajectories have attempted to understand how ordinary people navigate between therapeutic logics. However, in Keru, the ambiguity of care is not so much about choosing between therapeutic logics but about being open and taking advantage of the available options. By seeking and trying out different treatment options, mothers work hard to address both acute sicknesses and a fragile future. As Stacey Langwick points out in her study on the relationship between malaria and *degedege* in Tanzania: "The use of a therapy does not necessarily indicate faith in that therapy (or in the person administering it)" (Langwick 2007: 112). Studying the actual therapeutic (and preventive) practices (see also Mogensen 2005; Whyte 1997) allows us to better understand the importance of tending social relationships with both the representatives of the state and the non-human beings of the surrounding bush.

I sympathize with Clare Chandler and Uli Beisel's point (2017) that if we want to understand how a disease is enacted and managed in places with fragile health care systems, we need to not only concentrate on clinics and hospitals but also trace how therapeutic practices tally with treatment by local healers and with self-treatment within the household. Chandler and Beisel insist that "as social scientists, we have to pay attention to both: the formal health care sciences and practice and informal and improvised practices that are part of juggling everyday life. These different ways to know, treat and heal disease have to be folded into each other" (Chandler and Beisel 2017: 415; Hinchliffe and Ward 2014).

In both types of vaccinations described here, relationships between the individual and society understood broadly are nursed. It is not the technology itself that defines the type of "citizenship" at stake, whether bio-citizenship that focuses on the relationship between the individual and the state or spatial citizenship that tends the relationship between the individual and the non-human beings living outside the domestic space (and locality). Rather, how the technology is practiced defines the type of belonging addressed by the therapy.

In this chapter, we have seen two forms of vaccination; many mothers make use of both practices for their children. As individuals, they are not necessarily informed about which specific diseases the public health care vaccination program addresses, but they take time to visit the dispensary for vaccinations at times when their children are not suffering from a disease. Likewise, they consult Mariam, a marabout, or a bonesetter for both preventive practice and treatment. They do not focus on specific epistemologies, and they do not demand specific causal explanations. Rather, their overall concern is to protect their children. By taking advantage of the available options, they confirm both biosocial citizenship, which authenticates their relationship to the state through signatures of belonging like prescriptions, finger-pricks, and vaccination cards, and spatial citizenship, which reinforces their relationships to the local spiritual world through signatures of belonging such as bodily scars and amulets.

Notes

1. I never fully understood this calculation, but 165 CFA [franc] divided by five is 33 (the number for boys is three), and 220 CFA [franc] divided by five is 44 (the number for girls is four). The division by five relates to an older money system. See (see Fainzang 1985b) for a discussion of the relationship between gender and the numbers three and four.
2. The nurses, for their part, express frustrations about the health-seeking practices of the local population. Hamidou, a nurse at the local dispensary in Keru, responded to a question about what he perceived as their main challenge: "It is the fact that people do not come early enough for consultation. We also have problems at the level of sensitization; we don't know if people don't understand or if they refuse to understand" (interview, 2015).
3. The number of circulating vaccine-derived poliovirus cases (cVDPC) has increased since 2019 because of disruptions in surveillance and immunization during the COVID-19 pandemic (Venkatesan 2022).

4. World Health Organization, "Global Immunization 1980–2019," The Global Health Observatory. Retrieved 14 October 2020 from https://www.who.int/gho/immunization/dtp3/en/.
5. Gavi, the Vaccine Alliance, "GAVI Factsheet for Burkina Faso 2018." Retrieved 25 February 2020 from https://www.gavi.org/programmes-impact/country-hub/africa/burkina-faso.
6. I discuss the "low utilization" of health services in Burkina Faso in more detail in chapter 5.
7. According to the World Health Organization (WHO), full immunization means that a child has received the BCG vaccine (to prevent tuberculosis), the measles vaccine, three doses of polio vaccine, and three doses of the DPT (diphtheria, tetanus, and pertussis) vaccine.
8. Citizens also encounter state representatives in other situations, for example, at road blocks where military or police control vehicles and passengers and sometimes ask for money.
9. Scarification or cicatrization denotes the cutting and raising of scars into which a substance such as charcoal is rubbed in order to create a permanent mark. Tattooing, in contrast, refers to puncturing the skin with a sharp instrument to insert a permanent pigment (Vaughan 2007).
10. A vast body of anthropological literature on bodily modifications analyzes the body as a boundary phenomenon. See, for example, Alfred Gell's detailed work on Pacific tattooing (Gell 1993; Schildkrout 2004). Masks, as a mark of culture, may also be interpreted as a second skin (see Mauss 2001; Levi-Strauss 1963).
11. I return to a description of Dr. Sorgho's home clinic in chapter 5.
12. According to Sylvie Fainzang, the word "zina" originally derives from the Arabic word "djinna" or "jinn," but is integrated into the local Bissa cosmology (Fainzang 1986: 26).
13. Here, a fetish usually consists of two jars turned upside down.
14. I have not looked here at the many other technologies of the self that are used within the household, which is by far the most important place for health care activities (see chapter 2 for an in-depth discussion of care work and care practices in relation to small children).

Chapter 5
Treatment Seeking and the Work of Hope

In this chapter, I return to my initial queries when starting fieldwork in Keru concerning the use of public health care facilities. Are the facilities in rural areas underutilized? How is the relationship between rural citizens and the government health care system negotiated in everyday life? What is at stake? How has treatment seeking changed over the last couple of decades? How do mothers of sick children navigate between the so-called traditional and public therapeutic options? The village of Keru is my starting point, the place I have returned to, again and again, for almost twenty-five years. My analysis of the health system and care-seeking processes therefore also begins in this village. I look at the local dispensary (Centre de Santé et de Promotion Sociale) and the district hospital from the outside, from the perspective of its users (and non-users) rather than from the perspectives of the staff or government.

Taking this approach is, in a sense, to go against the contemporary trend among medical anthropologists, where the focus is on biomedicine and the clinic or hospital serves as the main field site (Hannig 2017; Livingston 2012; McKay 2017; Melberg, Diallo, Tylleskär, et al. 2016; Scherz 2018; Strong 2020; Wendland 2010). "Hospital ethnography" (Van der Geest and Finkler 2004; Long, Hunter, and Van der Geest 2008) has contributed tremendously to our understanding of biomedical institutions as porous and liminal places embedded in their surroundings (Hannig 2017: 9). These studies have enriched our understanding of a globalized medical economy. Through numerous fine-grained analyses of biomedical routines and procedures, as well as detailed studies of new medical technologies, we have seen how "local" biomedical institutions serve as places of entanglement (Gammeltoft 2014; Livingston 2012; McKay 2017; Mol 2002; Street 2012; Wahlberg and Gammeltoft 2018). However, as China Scherz contends, "We need scholarship that describes not only what happens to the few who [are] caught up in the biotechnical embrace, but also what happens to the people whose quests for therapy lie primarily outside of it" (2018: 548).[1]

This chapter speaks to the call of Vincanne Adams, Nancy J. Burke, and Ian Whitmarsh for slow research that "takes the local as the starting point" (2014: 181); my long-term engagement with one particular village is "slow" in a concrete, temporal sense, taking place over more than two decades. My aim is not necessarily to investigate whether the licensed health care workers are performing well, nor is it to question whether individual therapeutic trajectories are sound or rational. Rather, I seek to provide an understanding of the complex medical field, where citizens consult biomedical public health facilities and traditional practitioners in ways that are often nonsystematic, pragmatic, and tactical.

I begin with a brief overview of how the public health care system is organized in Burkina Faso, including a short introduction to the local dispensary in Keru.[2] From there, I discuss the main priorities of Burkina's health policy since the signing of the Alma Ata Declaration in 1978 in order to contextualize the services provided at the public clinics. I examine how mothers of sick children navigate the medical field, which, in addition to the public dispensary, includes a number of specialized healers as well as a very popular retired nurse, Dr. Sorgho, who provides biomedically based treatments to local residents. I ask whether the public health care system is underutilized through a discussion of the absent-present services provided at the local dispensary and of the mothers' pragmatic health-seeking practices (Whyte 1997). I argue that the process of seeking health care is about creating possibilities and about hope (Huskey 2009; Whyte 2005). In this part of the world, where child sickness is part of everyday life in a very literal sense and where health emergencies are chronic, health-seeking processes are about hoping for something and about living in hope. At every step, mothers hope for recovery and live in hope, reconciling themselves to an everyday life where children fall ill again and again.

Public Health Care in Burkina Faso

The mortality rate of children under five in Burkina Faso has declined dramatically over the last couple of decades, from 192.5 per thousand live births in 1996 to 87.5 in 2019.[3] This is an impressive achievement, explained primarily by increased healthcare seeking and improved malaria treatment (M. Ouédraogo et al. 2020; Sarrassat et al. 2019). However, poverty-related diseases continue to be widespread, with malaria, respiratory infections, and diarrheal diseases as the most common among children (UNICEF 2019: 10). In addition, malnutrition and stunting are widespread. While the mean life expectancy has increased over the last twenty years to around sixty-one years, it is still very low compared to most other countries.[4]

The public health care system in Burkina Faso is organized hierarchically with six main hospitals at the top, followed by medical centers and dispensaries. The country is divided into seventy health districts with a total of 2,126 Centres de Santé et de Promotion Sociale (CSPS), the dispensaries that provide primary health care (Ministère de la Santé 2022). The government of Burkina Faso has prioritized increasing the number of dispensaries in order to bring health care closer to the population and improve the quality of care at the peripheral level (Ministère de la Santé 2011). However, as I discuss in chapter 6, weak infrastructure and limited diagnostic capacity at the dispensaries challenge the system's ability to provide basic services to the rural population. The dispensaries, each of which covers an average of 9,332 people (Ministère de la Santé 2022: 60), are typically the entry point to the health care system, though outpatient departments at the medical centers and the district hospitals may also serve as the first contact. With empty rooms, scanty diagnostic equipment, and limited professional capacity, the dispensaries are instantiations of an "absent-present" state (Law 2002; Street 2014). The health staff at the dispensaries may refer patients to the higher levels of the health system, but ambulance services are scarce, so patients usually have to find their own transportation. Most of Burkina Faso's health care system is public, with some private facilities, a few of which are faith based, located primarily in urban areas. Various types of traditional healers, including herbalists, marabouts, bonesetters, and diviners, offer health care as part of the folk sector (Kleinman 1980), and self-treatment is also widespread (Gnawali et al. 2009; Østergaard, Bjertrup, and Samuelsen 2016; Samuelsen 2004a).

The Local Dispensary

The public dispensaries in Keru and Tenga are important sites for seeking health care, but they are often not the initial choice for treatment. The question about the extent to which government facilities are used opens up a broader discussion about people's experiences and expectations as well as about different forms of capital. From the perspective of the individual citizen of Keru, there are quite a few therapeutic options to choose between. In this particular locality, the medical field includes, in addition to the public biomedical institutions, a number of specialized health care practitioners,[5] including an assortment of part-time healers and herbal specialists, who in most cases address a narrow selection of specific symptoms or diseases. In addition, people commonly treat themselves or family members at home using herbs collected in the surrounding bush or using medicines, herbal medicine, or pharmaceutical products bought at the local market. The therapeutic trajectories of my interlocutors show that public health care facilities, such as the dispensary and the outpatient department at the nearest hospital, are not necessarily selected as the primary service providers.

The dispensary in Keru, which is supposed to be the first level of contact with the public health care system, was constructed in 2006 through the initiative of a well-off son of the village, who financed the construction and engaged a French NGO to build the facility. Despite the private donation, the dispensary was always part of the public health care system. Until the construction of this facility, the dispensary in Tenga, a village about four kilometers from Keru, served as the first-line public health care facility. Each of the ten dispensaries in the district serves ten to twelve villages with a total population of about 10,000 (as of 2015).[6]

The main dispensary building in Keru is a light yellow, square structure with a small patio containing a single bench where patients can wait. Two barred windows provide light and ventilation to the waiting room, which is separated from the patio by a wide entrance. The other windows of this main building are open frames covered with light blue metal slats. The cement floor and the lower half of the walls inside the patio are painted brown, and the upper walls are painted light yellow. A small copper sign above the main entrance mentions the private donor and the year of construction. Because of the climate, buildings in Burkina Faso quickly look dilapidated and in need of new paint, and this is certainly the case here, where the main dispensary building, despite its relatively recent construction, looks neglected. The outer walls, marked by dark blotches, bear the brunt of the infrequent but heavy rainfalls during the rainy season. The waiting room inside the main building is large and rather dark with a few metal benches in the middle. A few tatty posters with messages about the importance of getting one's children vaccinated and with instructions about how to use bed nets are pasted on the walls.

The consultation office is located on the right side of the waiting room; it is furnished with a wooden desk and two metal chairs, one for the nurse and one for the patient. A metal cabinet with old register books and other paperwork is placed in the corner, and a scale for weighing people is the only visible examination tool. A few rooms for admitted patients are also located inside the main building, each furnished with four or five metal beds with thin plastic mattresses placed along the walls in the otherwise empty rooms. Because treatment facilities are limited, few patients are admitted here, so very often these rooms are empty. Patients may be admitted at night when transport to hospital facilities is difficult or in cases where the nurse on duty decides that a patient needs to be observed for a day or two.

One early afternoon when I passed by to say hello to the nurse, I was met by the assistant nurse outside the dispensary informing me that the *matronne*, the head nurse, was busy with a patient in the consultation room. This was easy to hear, as a child was crying intensely and the voice of the nurse questioning the child's mother could be clearly heard above the crying. There were no other patients around that afternoon. Between the main building and a more recently constructed maternity section, there is a small house containing the medical depot. A village volunteer administers the medical depot under the responsibility of a local steering committee known as the Comité Gestion, or CoGes.[7] Pharmaceuticals are ordered through the district hospital using the Essential Drug List developed by the Ministry of Health and the World Health Organization (WHO). The volunteer in charge of the medical depot was a young woman who had organized the medical products neatly on the shelves behind the counter in the small room with a price list hanging on the wall. Patients come with prescriptions they have received from the nurse during their consultation. They collect the medicine, and, if the medical product is not exempt from payment, pay for it. The patients then return to the nurse in the consultation room for further instructions and injections, if prescribed.[8]

A maternity section was added to the facility in 2009. This separate building, which is painted rose and gray, is located just opposite the main consultation building. It consists of four or five rooms, including an office for the nurse, a delivery room, an admission room, and a storeroom, where supplementary food for malnourished children is stocked. The delivery room is equipped with a couple of delivery tables (one of which has stirrups), buckets for water, a baby-weighing scale, a tray with scissors and other instruments, and an autoclave to sterilize equipment. Official posters with health messages as well as handwritten procedural guidelines for health staff hang on the walls. A fine layer of red dust covers most surfaces in all of the buildings, and all the posters hanging on the walls have crumpled corners; perhaps this is due to the dry weather or how long they have been hanging there. While the maternity section clearly looks newer and perhaps also marginally better equipped, the absence of diagnostic tools, running water, and stable electricity is still remarkable.

The location of the dispensary in Keru and the fact that housing is provided for the nurses implies, at least in principle, the presence and availability of services 24/7. However, the dispensary was often remarkably empty with few, if any, patients. During most afternoons, the health staff were not present at the facility either. This is not to say that the nurses posted at the facility were not doing their jobs or that they were not performing well. They may have had very good reasons to leave the dispensary during the afternoons to attend training sessions or meetings. Seen from the outside, however, rural dispensaries generally seem to lack diagnostic equipment and adequate facilities, and absenteeism also seems common, as scholars studying rural health care facilities in other parts of the world have also noted (Banerjee and Duflo 2006; Nyamweya et al. 2017).

The next level of the health care system is the Centre Medical (Medical Center). Medical centers are usually equipped like the dispensary but include a medical doctor and sometimes a midwife and a laboratory technician, if there is a laboratory. The third and fourth levels of the health system are the district hospital and the regional hospital respectively. As there was no medical center near Keru, villagers would, in acute cases, if they managed to organize transport, go directly to the nearest specialized health care facility, the regional hospital, thereby skipping the levels of medical centers and district hospital. However, they were bureaucratically assigned to the district hospital, which was usually staffed with physicians, assistant doctors (*attachés de santé*), midwives, and nurses, as well as laboratory technicians and pharmacy staff. Very complicated cases would be referred to the university hospital in Ouagadougou.

Health Policy in Burkina Faso

A fundamental pillar of Burkina Faso's health care policy since independence is strong district-based primary health care. In 1978, the government signed the Alma Ata Declaration on Primary Health Care, a groundbreaking document that shaped health care policies globally during the following decades and that continues to inform policy in most sub-Saharan countries, including Burkina Faso, which signed the declaration only eighteen years after independence. The Alma Ata Declaration defines primary health care as follows:

> Primary health care is essential health care based on practical, scientifically sound and socially acceptable methods and technology made universally accessible to individuals and families in the community through their full participation and at a cost that the community and country can afford to maintain at every stage of their development in the spirit of self-reliance and self-determination. It forms an integral part both of the country's health system, of which it is the central function and main focus, and of the overall social and economic development of the community. It is the first level of contact of individuals, the family and community with the national health system bringing health care as close as possible to where people live and work, and constitutes the first element of a continuing health care process.[9]

The commitment to the Alma Ata Declaration implied that Burkina Faso, as well as the other 133 countries that signed it, now had to focus on providing basic health care services at the community level, making primary health care central in the overall structure of health care systems (Rifkin 2018). The government of Burkina Faso has since then worked quite intensely to increase the number of dispensaries in rural areas (Ministère de la Santé 2011). While the introduction of user fees increased resources for primary health care during the structural adjustment period of the 1990s, it also increased inequality, further excluded the poorest segment of the population, and increased poverty in an already impoverished population (Haddad, Nougtara, and Fournier 2006).

In the beginning of this chapter, I asked whether the public dispensaries in Keru and Tenga are "underutilized." I want to explain here what I mean by that. If we look at child health reports for Burkina Faso, we see improvements over the years. Child mortality rates decreased from 199 per thousand live births in 1990 to 87.5 in 2019 and 48 per thousand in 2021 (ICF, INSD 2022). This is a huge reduction, but the figures are still high compared to Burkina's neighbor Ghana, for example, where the under-five mortality rate was 30.8 per thousand live births in 2021.[10] According to UNICEF, although more children are surviving in Burkina, they are not necessarily thriving, and about 28 percent of children under five in the country are not growing well.[11] As discussed in other parts of this book, it is difficult to obtain valid statistics about symptoms and diseases that are not treated in the professional health care sector (Pierre Ilboudo, Chou, and Huang 2012), but UNICEF estimates that in Burkina Faso only around 50 percent of children with symptoms of acute respiratory infections seek treatment at a health care facility (UNICEF 2019). Other studies confirm that although health care services are available in Burkina Faso, they are not necessarily accessible. Jean-Louis Koulidiati and colleagues (2018) found that wealthier households used dispensary services more frequently and that the availability of staff in the dispensary also influenced their use. As we shall see below, my fieldwork observations confirm that many cases of child illness are cared for outside of the professional health sector.

In 2021, the primary level of the health care system in Burkina included 2,126 public dispensaries (CSPS). The average distance from an individual's home to the local health facility has been reduced from 9.8 km in 2001 to 6.1 km in 2021, though the average distance varies across different parts of the country (Ministère de la Santé 2011, 2022). In 1992, one CSPS served an average population of 13,230; by 2021 it had been reduced to an estimated 10,113 (Ministère de la Santé 2022). The availability of public health services in rural areas increased considerably over the last couple of decades, but studies show that the use of those facilities remains relatively low; that is also true in the province of Boulgou, where my fieldwork took place. Aude Meunier (1999) documented a decline in the use of public primary health care facilities in Houet Province over the five-year period from 1990 to 1995. Likewise, Valéry Ridde and colleagues (2013) report that the number of new contacts at the primary health care facilities per individual per year was 0.50 in 2008, only a slight increase from 0.40 in 1982. The number of new contacts started to increase after 2008, and by 2018, the Ministry of Health reported 1.22 contacts per inhabitant per year, with 3.09 contacts per year for children under five years of age (Ministère de la Santé 2019). However, more recent data show that this figure has fallen again to an average of 2.6 new contacts per year (Ministère de la Santé 2022).[12] As discussed elsewhere in this book, the absence of diagnostic equipment and staff absenteeism continue to challenge both the demand for public health care as well as the quality of health care services, particularly in rural areas.

In 2001, Burkina signed the Abuja Declaration, in which the heads of state of the African Union pledged, among other things, to allocate 15 percent of their annual budget to the health sector (WHO 2011). Later studies have shown that only Tanzania managed to live up to this ambitious goal. Burkina Faso is among a large group of countries that have made "insufficient progress," according to a WHO report evaluating results ten years after the declaration was signed (WHO 2011: 2). According to Burkina Faso's own national health statistics, about 13.5 percent of the government's budget was used on health in 2021, still below the original goal of 15 percent.

Burkina Faso also participated in other global goal-setting efforts. For example, the Millennium Development Goals were approved by a total of 189 countries, including Burkina Faso. However, the collection of data on the various indicators of this hugely ambitious plan to lift millions of people out of extreme poverty has been insufficient. The fact that Burkina Faso is praised for its progress toward achieving Target 1B—"full and productive employment and decent work for all, including women and young people" (Azevedo 2017: 75–76)—may incline one to ask questions about the validity of

Burkina's data, and the Ministry of Health itself expresses concerns about the quality of the routine data collected for the national health surveillance system. In one of the regular epidemiological bulletins issued by the Ministry of Health, the quality issue is addressed in an editorial: "One of the frequently mentioned reasons, when justifying the low quality of data, is the insufficient competence of the actors, who are responsible for the collection and reporting of data at the different levels of the health system. Lack of training of these people in how the Health Information System works and a lack of interest in providing good data quality contribute to the poor data quality" (Ministère de la Santé 2018:1). National health policy documents and declarations include a number of detailed, quantifiable targets, particularly in relation to mother-child health care. At the same time, everyone, including the Ministry of Health, seems to know that these goals are built on weak and often disputable data (Adams 2016; Erikson 2016; Jerven 2013; Tichenor 2017). In chapter 6, I discuss the increasing significance of data and statistics at the national and international levels in more detail.

In the preamble of the National Health Care Policy covering the period from 2011 to 2020, the minister of health highlighted the government's commitment to work toward the Sustainable Development Goals, particularly goals aimed at reducing infant mortality, improving maternal health, and fighting HIV/AIDS, malaria, and other diseases. In the second paragraph of this preamble, the minister emphasized Burkina's commitment to the Abuja Declaration's commitment to spend at least 15 percent of the government's budget on the health sector. He also highlighted the country's commitment to the 2008 Ouagadougou Declaration, which emphasizes a strengthening of primary health care and health systems in Africa (Ministère de la Santé 2011).

Since independence in 1960, the government of Burkina Faso has attuned its health care policy and strategic plans to various international and regional declarations and to the recommendations of the WHO. The strategic plans have all focused on improving mother and child health, strengthening primary health care, and addressing the country's heavy malaria burden. A central element of health care policy throughout this period has been decentralizing the health care system and increasing the number of dispensaries, thus reducing the distance people have to travel to reach public health facilities. The emphasis on user fees during the period of structural adjustment in the 1990s hit poor communities hard. A more recent policy providing free treatment for children under five has probably increased the number of consultations, although "free" services and medicine are not always free. The national health policy of Burkina Faso continues to focus on primary health care, although the increased burden of chronic diseases (diabetes, cardiovascular diseases, and mental illness) is also mentioned as an important point for attention (Ministère de la Santé 2011).[13]

Utilization of the Public Dispensary

On most occasions when I passed by the rural dispensaries in Tenga and Keru, I remarked on how quiet and empty the facilities appeared. Whether the emptiness reflected low capacity or low demand by the rural communities (or both) was difficult to say. In chapter 6, I discuss this question in more detail. Here, I want to examine the use of health care facilities by looking at the facilities from the outside, from the point of view of local citizens and from my own observations. Over the past twenty years, everyday life in Keru, Tenga, and other villages in the province has changed in a number of ways: the population has more than doubled, a new dispensary has opened in Keru, more health care staff have been assigned, and some of the reporting procedures have changed.

The Demographic Health Surveys provide contextual information about the overall health care situation in the country, as well as about the use of the health care system.[14] Comparing specific data from three DHS reports—from 1998–1999, 2010, and 2021—highlights some important changes.[15] First, the proportion of rural residents remained high in 2010, with about 77 percent of the Burkinabe population living in rural areas, only a small drop from 1998–1999 (INSD 2012). In the 2021 report, it is estimated that 33 percent of females and 36 percent of males live in urban areas (ICF, INSD 2022). Furthermore, school attendance among females has remained very low during the whole period. The 1998–1999 report estimates that 83.9 percent of Burkinabe females never attended school; this dropped slightly to 78.7 percent in the 2010 report with a further drop to 58 percent in 2021. Education is often mentioned by public health experts as the most important indicator for whether people adhere to public health messages and participate in democratic processes (Katahoire et al. 2004; MacLean 2011).

Skilled birth attendance is often used as a proxy for quality of care, and rural women are increasingly turning to public health facilities for delivery. In the 1998–1999 report, 73.8 percent of rural women were giving birth at home. This figure dropped dramatically to 38.7 percent in 2010 and to about 7 percent in 2021. This shift could potentially lead to lower maternal mortality rates, though researchers question whether skilled birth attendance is a relevant proxy for quality of birth care (A. H. Diallo et al. 2010; Melberg, Diallo, Ruano, et al. 2016). The child vaccination program is, however, a clear success story. Children aged twelve to twenty-three months who have received all the recommended vaccinations increased from 26 percent in 1998–1999 to 81 percent in 2010, though it fell slightly to 79 percent in 2021 (ICF, INSD 2022: 34)

Over time, people in Burkina Faso have increasingly accessed public health care facilities in response to the most frequent childhood diseases. About 50 percent of children suffering from upper respiratory infections, fever, or diarrhea during the fourteen-day period prior to the surveys were brought for consultation at a health facility in 2010, an increase from about 20 percent in the 1998–1999 survey (DHS, MEASURE 2010; Institut National de la Statistique et de la Démographie 2000). In the 2022 report, the statistics are compiled a bit differently; here 80 percent of children under five with symptoms of upper respiratory infections were brought for consultation. The figures for fever and diarrhea were 75 percent and 63 percent respectively.[16]

Increasing use of public health facilities is to be expected, as the national health strategy has emphasized the importance of primary health care for decades. An increased number of consultations at government health care facilities does not, of course, speak to the quality of care or its outcome—that is, did the health of the patient actually improve? Besides, the facilities in Keru and Tenga continue to be characterized by absences: the absence of diagnostic equipment, the absence of staff (during many afternoons), and the absence of ambulances for referrals. The dispensary often looked empty in the afternoon, with no staff or just a single person, and with very few if any patients to care for. The dispensaries are busiest from August through October, the peak season for malaria. In addition, the dispensaries are quite busy on vaccination days—as mentioned, the vaccination rates, particularly in the rural regions, are very high.[17] Unfortunately, full information is lacking about disease burdens and the effectiveness of the services provided at the local dispensaries, which makes analyzing their use more difficult.

As the rest of this chapter shows, the use of government health facilities is just part of the story of healthcare seeking in rural Burkina Faso. Mothers navigate a medical field in which many different health care providers offer their services, and the mothers' individual pathways cross in and out of the public facilities in combination with home treatment and consultations with various local health care specialists. While other studies have documented similar health-seeking trajectories, my focus in this chapter adds a new perspective to my argument that rural citizens, particularly women responsible for the daily care of their children, work extremely hard to prevent, care, and treat childhood illnesses. It also shows that various healing traditions and professionalized practices are entangled with each other and demonstrates that, despite a political focus on improving the availability of primary health care, its accessibility and quality remains limited.

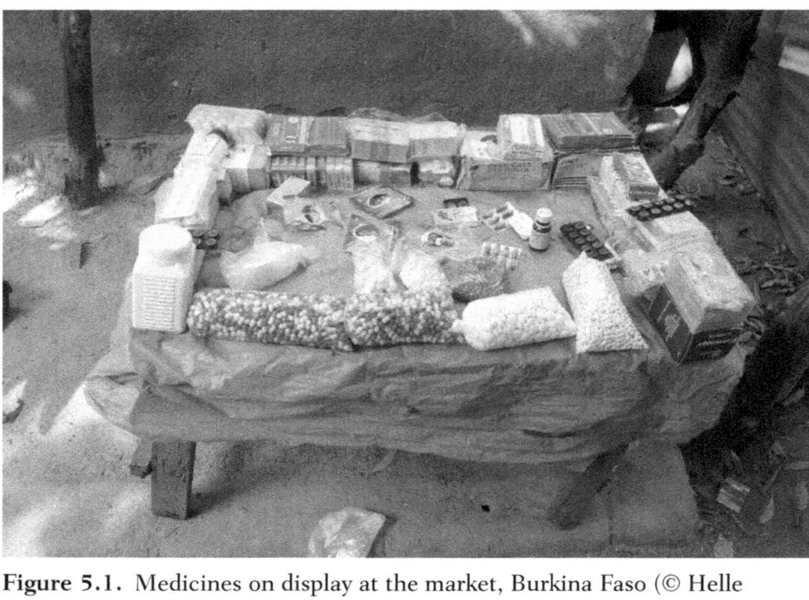

Figure 5.1. Medicines on display at the market, Burkina Faso (© Helle Samuelsen 2023)

Multiple Therapeutic Options

The disease pattern of the citizens of Keru might be much more complex than that reflected in the monthly reports from the local dispensary. The use of the local dispensary may reflect a "supply-driven" approach: most people in the village know that the nurses at the dispensary are able to diagnose malaria, and the medical depots usually have malaria medicine in stock, so the villagers go to the dispensary when they have symptoms associated with malaria. In other words, the villagers demand the services they know can be supplied.[18] However, as I realized during my very first time in the area, a number of other health care services are available.

I identified about twenty-five local people who offered some kind of health services. The majority were herbalists, who collect leaves, roots, and bark in the surrounding bush, prepare medicine, and treat villagers who turn up for consultation. Mariam Salemporgo, *la vaccinatrice*, whose practice I discussed in chapter 4, was one of these herbalists. Most of the herbalists, including Mariam, specialized in treating specific symptoms or diseases. Bonesetters, who had special skills in treating fractures, were consulted by local citizens with broken bones due to falling from trees or being injured in traffic. I also encountered Salif, a respected citizen of Keru, who specialized in addressing cases of sorcery. As far as I know, he was the only person in the village with these skills. Like most of the other healers, he spent most of his time doing farm work, tending his fields, only offering advice and treatment when villagers asked him to. On the periphery of Keru, a diviner who nursed special relations with the spirits of the bush lived alone in a small round mud-brick house. He was consulted not only in cases of sickness but also in response to other misfortunes. A number of marabouts, Islamic specialists who had acquired skills in treating sickness, used quotations from the Qur'an, sometimes in combination with other therapies based on herbs or minerals. Furthermore, I encountered Dr. Sorgho, who, upon his retirement as a public health care nurse, began to treat local residents from his home clinic.

The therapeutic skills of the vernacular healers are both technical and spiritual. While the technical skills include specific knowledge about certain plants and their use in treating specific symptoms, the spiritual skills, which are either inherited or in some cases acquired through a traumatic event or from religious texts, are as important for the success of the healing process (Fainzang 1986).

Dr. Sorgho

About a month into my first period of fieldwork in the area, I met Dr. Sorgho. I was visiting Bangri, a local village, in the company of Thomas, Beatrice (who carried their youngest son, Michel, on her back), and Jean. We had set out from Keru on foot in order to pay Beatrice's elderly mother a visit. Beatrice was raised in Bangri and had moved to Keru when she married Thomas. We walked the four or five kilometers from Keru to Bangri through a landscape of millet, sorghum, and corn fields intersected by areas of grass and thorny bushes. In some fields, the harvesting of sorghum had already started. It was the rainy season, but there had been no rain for a couple of days and the temperature was high. We had to cross a small river that is usually dry, but at this time of the year it was filled with water. Spirits were high, and we walked quickly. Beatrice did not want to get back to Keru too late, as she wanted to continue brewing millet beer for her *cabaret*, which would be open the following day.

After reaching Beatrice's mother's compound, we were seated outside on small benches and were immediately served fresh water. As custom prescribes, greetings and introductions take place after guests are seated and served something to drink, either water or *dolo*, the local millet beer. Thomas had brought a couple of kola nuts, which he passed on to his mother-in-law to pay his respects.[19] After a short conversation with Beatrice's family members, we moved on, passing a small marketplace where a few stalls were selling vegetables and everyday utensils. We then reached another big compound with a number of small houses inside. A large man dressed in what is sometimes called "colonial bureaucratic" dress—a uniform-like jacket and trousers in either khaki or, as in this case, dark green—was sitting in a chair under a *hangar* (shelter) wearing sunglasses and a huge gold watch. He was listening to a small radio playing scratchy music. A few young men hung around, sitting on small benches or piles of wood, making it obvious that this elderly man was important. Thomas introduced me to Dr. Sorgho. He welcomed me and asked if I liked *dolo*. After I confirmed politely that I did, Dr. Sorgho handed some coins to one of the young men, who immediately disappeared into the compound. A few minutes later, he came back with *dolo* in a four-liter plastic container—one that originally had been used for diesel—and a calabash to drink from, handing both to me. Of course, I could not drink four liters of *dolo* myself, but since I could not take the container with me, we had to finish it before moving on. We all shared it together while listening to the story of Dr. Sorgho.

Dr. Sorgho was born in the village of Bangri, and, after many years of service in the public health sector, had now returned to the village and set up a popular private clinic in his home. Dr. Sorgho was not trained as a physician but as a public health nurse. However, his patients and people in the surrounding villages always used the title "doctor." Likewise, nurses at the dispensary are often called doctors, and dispensaries are often called hospitals. During his career, Dr. Sorgho had been posted in various provinces as well as in the provincial town Tenkodogo. He was the first nurse employed at the dispensary in Tenga, a neighboring village, when it was established in the early 1990s.

His home clinic was not a clinic in any conventional sense: he simply sat inside his compound most days, with patients waiting every morning (except Sundays) outside under a *hangar*. One after another, patients were allowed into his compound for consultation. He was very popular, and people arrived early to be among the first in the long queue. His therapy was based exclusively on biomedicine, and he used to stock pharmaceuticals that he had purchased in town so that his patients could be treated immediately without having to search for medical products at the market. He did not have a refrigerator or cooling facilities, so he chose products that did not require refrigeration. He was relatively well-off, with well-educated sons, one of whom worked as a physician at a hospital in the capital, Ouagadougou. While his sons had moved away from the village, he had decided to move back after his retirement, a decision the local citizens both respected and appreciated.

His household was very large, with four wives and forty-two children, so the compound was full of small houses. Later, some of the small round mud-brick houses were replaced by larger square cement-brick houses, as seen in many villages where family members had done well as migrant workers, public servants, or entrepreneurs. His youngest wife, like Beatrice, ran a millet beer *cabaret* every third day. Most often he was wearing a colonial-style suit, typical of government officials, but sometimes he was dressed in a typical Burkinabe boubou, a wide-sleeved tunic very popular during the revolutionary period of Thomas Sankara, who promoted this "simple" cotton clothing for all Burkinabes to show their "ordinary humbleness." Its design, with a white background and blue, black, and white stripes, is still seen quite often in Burkina on both men and women.

During one of my early interviews with Thomas, he emphasized Dr. Sorgho's popularity as he explained the "everyday" trajectory for treating illness:

> *Thomas*: When a person is sick, we first try to treat with plants. If there are no improvements, then we go for consultation at the dispensary.
>
> *Helle*: Do you then go to the dispensary in Tenga?
>
> *Thomas*: Yes, we first buy medicine at the market here. If it does not work, then we go to Tenga. If they are out of stock, we sometimes go to Bangri to consult a retired nurse in order to buy medicines.
>
> *Helle*: Is he better than the nurses at the dispensary?
>
> *Thomas*: Yes, he is better, because he is a specialist. He is old, and he has a lot of experience.
>
> *Helle*: Does he charge you when you consult him?
>
> *Thomas*: No, he takes nothing. Everybody likes to consult him because he sometimes does us a favor. You consult him, and he prescribes, if he has the product, he treats you, and he gives you credit—you give him CFA [franc] 2,500 today, then tomorrow or after two or three days you give him CFA [franc] 3,000 or 3,500, like that. Even if you do not have money the first time, he treats you, and then you pay later. If you have money with you, you pay.
>
> *Helle*: And at the dispensary, you have to pay?
>
> *Thomas*: At the dispensary, after the consultation, they prescribe the medicines. It is when you go and buy the products that the treatment starts. That is why many prefer to consult the pensioned nurse, because he has the medicines, and he gives you a favor.

Injections were also very common in Dr. Sorgho's consultation, as they were at the local public health dispensary, and patients were often asked to come back in the afternoon or on the following day in order to complete their treatment (see also Birungi 1998; Birungi and Whyte 1994; Whyte, Van der Geest, and Hardon 2002). Interviews with seventeen patients consulting Dr. Sorgho on two consecutive days revealed that all were treated with injections. Apparently, the therapies and medicines prescribed by Dr. Sorgho and the nurses at the dispensary were very similar. Likewise, the prices for treatment at the two facilities seemed to be the same, but the queues were always longer at Dr. Sorgho's clinic. Below, I return to the issue of payment, which was definitely one of the reasons Dr. Sorgho was popular. But his popularity was also rooted in the simple fact that he was part of the local community: he was known and respected, and he knew almost everyone in his own village as well as in the nearest two or three other villages. Dr. Sorgho had worked at other locations, but he had come home. He could have settled comfortably in Ouagadougou or Tenkodogo with one or two of his wives, but he preferred to spend his last years in Bangri "doing something good for his own community," as people explained to me.

Dr. Sorgho linked state space with local space. He lived like most other villagers in this area, although his family was more educated and wealthier than most other local families. The architecture of his compound was the same as most other compounds, and his wife produced *dolo* for her *cabaret*, an institution firmly rooted in Bissa identity. He had adjusted his clinical practice to the local conditions by providing credit. On the other hand, he also represented a specific form of professionalism, similar to the one found within the public health system. He treated with pharmaceuticals only, a skill he had learned at the nursing school far from the village, which is associated with the European medical profession (*medicaments du blanc*). He took payment in cash rather than in kind, in contrast to local herbalists, who more commonly demanded a chicken or other food items in addition to small amounts of money. His manner of dress—sometimes "bureaucratic," sometimes "traditional"—associated him both with his former life as part of the government bureaucracy and with the local culture.

Forms of Capital

If we apply a Bourdieusian lens, the public dispensary and the many different local healers are agents in a medical field who position themselves and are positioned through the citizens' therapeutic trajectories. In Keru and the surrounding villages, we could map a field with a number of health care providers, each with their own specialization. As William Hanks emphasizes, fields should not be understood as conscious constructions or closed domains with explicit roles, but rather as a set of agents who invest in the field and struggle for the "reward" like participants in a game (Bourdieu 1990b; Hanks 1996). Each of the participants has a stake and an interest in the field. Pierre Bourdieu says:

> The existence of a specialized and relatively autonomous field is correlative with the existence of specific stakes and interests; via the inseparably economic and psychological investments that they arouse in the agents endowed with a certain habitus, the field and its stakes (themselves produced as such by relations that are constitutive of the field) produce investments of time, money and work, etc. In other words, interest is at once a condition of the functioning of a field (a scientific field, the field of haute couture, etc.) in so far as it is what "gets people moving," what makes them get together, compete and struggle with each other, and a product of the way the field functions. (Bourdieu 1990a: 87–88)

The medical field described here is a social space where different forms of capital play out and where the actual position in the field depends on the strength or value of the various forms of capital at a given time. In this particular context, it is clear that the public dispensaries in Keru and Tenga have a large amount of economic capital, as the movement of money and valuable goods is high, and the licensed health workers have regular salaries, unlike most villagers. To a certain extent, the health staff have symbolic capital through their position as government employees, who belong to the bureaucratic field and the field of power. Because of the rotation system, where most licensed health workers are attached to a specific health facility for a limited period, often two to four years, most of them, contrary to Dr. Sorgho, have little social capital in the community they serve. They are not permanent residents, they often belong to other ethnic groups, and, because they do not speak Mooré or Bissa, many of them face difficulties communicating with the local villagers.

Bourdieu's social analyses are often rightly criticized for being static and for neglecting the perspectives of the various agents or stakeholders. However, in this particular context, the medical field is useful as a way to map and position health care providers, as it offers a broader definition of the local system, including both public biomedical facilities and local healing traditions (Kleinman 1978; 1980; Samuelsen 2016; Strathern 1996). The notions of "field" and "game" emphasize how important social relations are in health care. This includes both the relationship between the individual health care provider and her "patient" as well as the relationships between providers. Occasionally, providers referred patients to each other (it was mostly the traditional healers who referred patients to the dispensary or directly to the hospital), but they were also very conscious about their own individual special skills or "gifts." They did not want to disclose their magic secrets to others.

In contrast to the licensed health workers, many of the herbalists had substantial cultural and social capital. With their practical and spiritual knowledge, they were able to nurture or restore the balance between the human and the spiritual worlds. Their families were grounded in the community; they shared their everyday life with other community members and participated in social events. In addition, the marabouts possessed cultural capital as they engaged in the production and reproduction of the moral world through their preventive, therapeutic, and religious practices. As skilled readers of the Qur'an, they were rich in cultural capital represented by the book itself, as well as by the pen, the board, the local medical products, and the amulets. As an educated, elderly, highly respected man

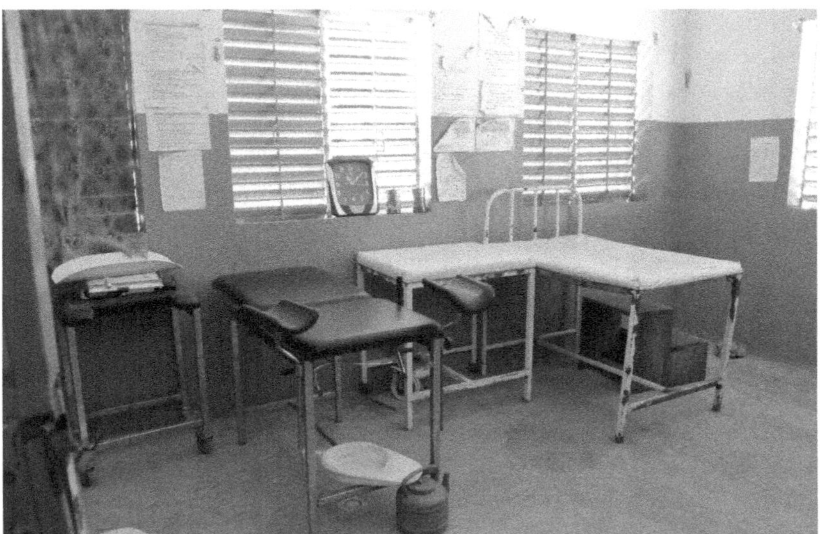

Figure 5.2. Examination room at a rural dispensary, Burkina Faso (© Helle Samuelsen 2023)

who had returned to his natal village to serve his community and offer them "favors" through his credit system, Dr. Sorgho possessed all forms of capital within the medical field.

Navigating the Medical Field

As I explained in chapter 2, mothers' pathways to find healing for their children were seldom linear; they steered through the medical field based on a number of practical considerations, some of which I briefly illustrate here. *Yingwingre*,[20] which literally means "warm body" in Bissa, is one of the illnesses most often mentioned by mothers of small children. It is characterized by a feverish condition and often translated as *fievre* (Schieffelin et al. 2014) or *paludisme* (malaria) by my research assistants and local French-speaking people. *Yingwingre* may go on for weeks, often in combination with other symptoms. As shown above, mothers often began treatment by departing for the bush to find specific leaves, roots, or bark, which they brought home and prepared as treatment for their sick child.

Daritou, a young mother with a six-month-old baby, explained that she used leaves from two different trees, *siiga* and *bagunde*. She boiled the leaves, then washed and purged the child with the liquid morning and evening. She continued this treatment for a couple of days, and if it did not reduce the symptoms, she then consulted the dispensary. Safia, another young woman in Keru, took various actions to treat her daughter, who suffered from *yingwingre* and *woubgo* (vomiting). During the first few days of sickness, she went to the dispensary and also treated her child at home with herbal products. At the dispensary, the child received an injection in addition to a prescription for medicine. Based on advice from an old woman living in the neighborhood, Safia collected leaves from three different trees, which she boiled, cooled, and gave the child to drink; she also washed him in the liquid until he was well again. Odette, a mother of seven children, did not use traditional medicine for *yingwingre*; instead, she went directly to the dispensary, as she explained: "The local medicine does not cure the disease completely. Consulting a *guerisseur* (herbalist) takes a lot of time. It is better and faster to go directly to the dispensary."

The treatment-seeking processes of Daritou, Safia, and Odette were characterized by pragmatic considerations: availability, accessibility, time, cost, and previous experience. The many treatment-seeking itineraries I encountered in Keru and neighboring villages show that mothers listened to advice from family members and neighbors, and with patience they seized opportunities for treatment based on their reading of the symptoms and on their individual constraints and possibilities for maneuvering within the medical field.

Hoping

Consulting the local dispensary was just one option among others for mothers of sick children in rural Burkina—and in many cases it was not the first option. A range of factors shaped treatment decisions. Some women had to ask their husband for approval before going to a health facility, particularly if it required payment (and it often did, even if treatment of children under five was, in principle, free). Moreover, previous experiences with particular healers influenced mothers' decisions, as did advice from family or community members. Furthermore, certain diseases were generally treated only at the biomedical facilities, while others were treated only by one of the local healers.

In chapter 2, I examined the relationship between mothers and their small children, particularly during periods of sickness. Inspired by Paul Ricoeur (1994), I focused on their practical care work as well as their treatment seeking. Here, I discuss how mothers navigate through the medical field in their relentless efforts to keep their children healthy. Mothers spent an incredible amount of time seeking treatment for their children. At each step in the process, they hoped for improvement, despite their past experience that the child, after improving, could easily relapse into sickness again, or another child might fall ill. They acted flexibly, reflecting a pragmatic recognition of the uncertainties they faced: "Here, when your child is sick you pray and ask God to give good health. You also find leaves, boil them, and wash the child with that. It may work, or it may not work. If it doesn't, you will bring the child to the health care center. And if the child doesn't get better, you will return to prayers" (quoted in Østergaard, Bjertrup, and Samuelsen 2016: 6).

The mothers' flexible route between healers and health care facilities was saturated with uncertainties and hope (Whyte 2005). As Nauja Kleijst and Stef Jansen (2016) remind us, "Uncertainty is a precondition for hope." Illness is a process in time, where treatment is pursued and recovery is hoped for. As with any other hope, the hope connected to treatment seeking is also about the future (Hage 2016). Ricoeur defines hope as a capacity concerned with seeking some good: "The act of hoping is an act which moves me in the direction of the desired good" (Huskey 2009: 27). It is not about passivity, where one waits for others to bring that which is searched for. Ricoeur argues that hope is active and implies action. The care work of rural mothers in Burkina is work of hope. Their "make do" pragmatic and tactical actions are directed toward sustaining the health of their children and improving their everyday life. Ricoeur, like Søren Kierkegaard, recognizes the fragility of hope. "Hope does not reconcile," Ricoeur says, "but rather consoles" (in Huskey 2009: 30). The mothers' therapeutic trajectories revealed a tension between hoping for something, that is, hoping that each consultation or treatment would result in the recovery of the child, and living in hope, that is, reconciling themselves to an everyday life subject to recurrent episodes of sickness among their children (Benzein, Norberg, and Saveman 2001; Huskey 2009).

The Money Issue

Several times in this chapter I have mentioned the cost of treatment. In a poor society like Burkina Faso, where most people live from subsistence agriculture, the amount of cash circulating is quite low. This was particularly the case during my first periods of fieldwork; now, because of remittances from family members, the flow of money has increased. However, with very few salaried workers and unpredictable remittances, family income is rarely stable. In addition, women, who traditionally take care of household matters including fetching wood, washing clothes, cooking, and taking care of small children and other family members in need, were even less likely to have cash. Their chance of securing a separate income was low, though some women sold vegetables from their gardens, sold food at market days, or organized a *cabaret*, as Beatrice did. If a woman managed to get an income, she usually had the right to keep the money for herself, which in reality meant that she had some money to pay for medicine or clothes for her children.

A visit to a health facility or a traditional healer almost always implied expenses, and all—and here I mean literally all the women I encountered during fieldwork—talked about the high cost of health care. This observation is confirmed by the 2010 Demographic Health Survey, in which 76.3 percent of rural women surveyed said they experience payment as an obstacle for consultations at the government health care facilities (DHS, MEASURE 2010). Treatment of children under five years of age has been free at the facilities since 2016. While this has been a huge benefit for poor households in urban as well as rural areas, it has also caused new uncertainties, as the supply of medicines to the rural dispensaries has been irregular. When medicines are absent, health staff have to ask patients, or parents of a sick child, to find the prescribed medicine themselves at a pharmacy in town or at the village market. Thomas explained: "If they don't have the products [at the dispensary], the parents have to pay. If they don't do that, the child will die. The parents complain, saying that the treatment is supposed to be free. But you have to go and buy the products and return [to the dispensary] to get your child treated. Often, they don't have the medicines. They only give out paracetamols, the rest you have to buy yourself." This may be embarrassing to parents who had not anticipated the potential extra cost. In addition, it created uncertainties about whether to try out other treatments before contacting the dispensary or whether to use the dispensary at all. These uncertainties complicated the treatment-seeking process.

In my experience, rural citizens carefully considered the various options for treating illness. Many mothers of sick children told me that they constantly worried about both the direct and indirect costs of treatment. Because of the high frequency of illness, each time they had to balance the question of what would be the most adequate treatment with the question of what would be the best to do in this case of sickness at this moment in time. Delphine, whose husband had been in Equatorial Guinea for six years, said that she either used herbal medicine or consulted the dispensary when any of her five children had fallen sick, saying: "For the last six years, I have taken care and paid for medications when they are sick. I also sell my animals to treat children in case of illness." Delphine was farming the family land, like so many other women staying behind, while her husband was on a migratory *aventure*. Decisions about what to do in cases of illness were always ambiguous, and although Delphine was in regular contact with her husband, it was difficult for her to make ends meet, as she explained: "He used to send [money], but since he started building his house, we don't get any money anymore except when Christmas is approaching. If he's sending money, it will be for next Christmas. If there are expenses in the family, I bear them." In other words, consulting the rural dispensary is an option for mothers, but uncertainties about how much it will cost and how to find the money mean that it may not necessarily be the first choice (Østergaard, Bjertrup, and Samuelsen 2016: 7).

As mentioned above, Dr. Sorgho's home clinic was very popular, in part because he provided credit. Based on the patients I interviewed, the average cost for pharmaceuticals at his clinic was similar to that of the public health dispensary. The kind of medicines and the therapies prescribed for patients were also very similar. However, Dr. Sorgho always started treatment immediately and did not request payment from his patients until the treatment was finished; even then, he often extended credit. Patients could stretch the payment over several months according to their individual financial situation. Almost all of his patients paid in installments, and he claimed that more than 90 percent of his patients eventually paid for their treatment. In contrast, the staff at the public health dispensary was not formally allowed to offer credit.

Conclusion

In this chapter, I demonstrate that although the rural residents in this part of Burkina Faso had access to public health care facilities located in their community, they navigated among multiple local health care providers. Their *metis*, their practical sense, made them move between treating illness at home, purchasing pharmaceuticals at the local market, and consulting various specialists, of which the public health nurse at the dispensary was but one. Since the signing of the Alma Ata Declaration, the government of Burkina Faso has prioritized mother-child health care services and the fight against malaria; however, this chapter demonstrates that caring for sick children is ambiguous and continues to encumber the everyday life of mothers in Keru and neighboring communities. Easy access to primary health care services has been a main priority for the government of since independence, and data suggest that the number of visits at the public health facilities has increased over time. Distance to a health facility is certainly an important factor for utilization, but the absent-present nature of these services places them as just one option among many in a medical field, where health care providers possess varying forms of capital. Uncertainties and lack of transparency about cost of treatment—despite an official user-fee policy and payment exemptions for children under five—play a huge role in everyday therapeutic pathways. Dr. Sorgho, the pensioned nurse who had set up his private home clinic in Bangri, offered credit to his patients, a gesture that made him extremely popular in the local community.

The historical and economic context of the health care system in Burkina Faso is important to consider. The system is underfinanced and structurally weak: the country spends only about US$40 on health per capita,[21] very little compared to most other countries in the world. In addition, part of this spending is diluted by corruption that takes place at all levels of the health care system (REN-LAC 2018). Caring for sick children continues to be a time-consuming part of everyday life in this part of Africa. Mothers zigzag between different types of specialists, hoping that each visit will result in improved health and living in hope as they strive for a good life.

Notes

1. This point was also made by Arthur Kleinman in his presentation about the three sectors (the professional sector, the folk sector, and the popular sector), in which he pointed out that most health care practices take place in the popular sector (Kleinman 1980). In this chapter, I use Kleinman's definition of the professional sector as the licensed and institutionalized health care services that are recognized by the state and have a monopoly on certain kinds of treatment.
2. In order to maintain anonymity, I do not describe the precise location of Keru or the specific health facilities mentioned in this chapter.
3. World Bank, "Mortality rate, under-5 (per 1,000 live births)—Burkina Faso." Retrieved 17 July 2023 from https://data.worldbank.org/indicator/SH.DYN.MORT?locations=BF.
4. UNICEF, "The State of the World's Children 2019 Statistical Tables," October 2019. Retrieved 17 July 2023 from https://data.unicef.org/resources/dataset/sowc-2019-statistical-tables.
5. In chapter 4, I discussed the practices of the local *vaccinatrice* and a number of marabouts and bonesetters.
6. These figures were provided by the district medical officer during an interview in 2015. In 2021, the number of dispensaries has increased to fourteen, each serving a population of around 10,000 (Ministère de la Santé 2022).

7. Each dispensary has a CoGes (Comité Gestion) that includes male and female community members (Sombié et al. 2017).
8. The policies for user fees and eligibility for free health care have changed quite a lot over the years.
9. The International Conference on Primary Health Care, "Declaration of Alma-Ata." Retrieved 17 July 2023 from https://cdn.who.int/media/docs/default-source/documents/almaata-declaration-en.pdf?sfvrsn=7b3c2167_2.
10. Macrotrends, "Ghana Infant Mortality Rate 1950–2023." Retrieved 17 July 2023 from https://www.macrotrends.net/countries/GHA/ghana/infant-mortality-rate.
11. UNICEF, "The State of the World's Children 2019." Retrieved 17 July 2023 from https://www.unicef.org/documents/state-of-worlds-children-2019-regional-briefs.
12. The decrease in 2020 and 2021 may be related to the COVID-19 pandemic.
13. A new national health policy was under development during 2021, but in early 2023, the official website of the Ministry of Health (Ministère de la Santé) continued to refer to the health strategy of 2011: *Plan National De Developpement Sanitaire 2001–2010*. Retrieved 17 July 2023 from https://www.sante.gov.bf/fileadmin/user_upload/storages/fichiers/plan_national_de_developpement_sanitaire.pdf.
14. The Demographic Health Surveys (DHS) are conducted by Macro International in collaboration with the Institut National de la Statistique et de la Démographie (INSD), Burkina Faso.
15. The 2010 DHS report is the most recent full report. A 2020 report was planned, and although data collection could not take place in all parts of Burkina Faso due to the security situation, a report with key indicators came out in July 2022 (ICF, INSD 2022).
16. In the 1998–1999 DHS survey, only consultations for upper respiratory infections and diarrhea were registered, not consultations for fever. In the 2021 survey, data for the three types of symptoms were registered separately, and the number of consultations increased for all three.
17. It is interesting to note that women are particularly invested in the vaccination programs, bringing their babies to the facilities at moments when their children are not sick.
18. I take up this discussion in more detail in chapter 6.
19. Kola nuts are a very bitter nut that is grated and held in the mouth. The juice from the nut has a stimulating effect like coffee. Traditionally, kola nuts are given to elderly people or people with greater status as a way to show respect.
20. Bissa words are spelled in many different ways. *Yingwingre* is also sometimes spelled "Yin-Wingre."
21. World Bank, "Current Health Expenditure Per Capita (current US$)—Afghanistan, Burkina Faso." Retrieved 17 July 2023 from https://data.worldbank.org/indicator/SH.XPD.CHEX.PC.CD?locations=AF-BF&most_recent_value_desc=false.

Part III

Care of the Public

Chapter 6
The Availability Logic

Every month, the nurses in charge of the dispensaries in Tenga and Keru have to submit a report to the district health authorities with information about the services provided during the previous month. These reports are preformatted with a number of tables based on the World Health Organization's International Statistical Classification of Diseases and Related Health Problems (ICD).[1] More than forty different diagnoses are listed on the form. Careful reading of the monthly reports from the two dispensaries showed that the diagnosis of *paludisme simple* (uncomplicated malaria) accounted for a very large proportion of the "new consultations," and the proportion increased over the years—for example, from 28.4 percent of all cases at the health center in Tenga in 2001 to 46.4 percent in 2013. At the dispensary in Keru, the malaria diagnosis was applied in more than half of all new consultations in 2010 and 2013—even in January, which is not the peak season for malaria.

Malaria is considered endemic in large parts of West Africa, including Burkina Faso. As the health facilities in Tenga and Keru observed an increase in registered malaria cases, the world experienced a rapid decline. As World Health Organization (WHO) director Margaret Chang explained in the foreword to the *World Malaria Report 2015*: "Our report tracks a dramatic decline in the global malaria burden over 15 years. Target 6C of the 2000 Millennium Development Goals called for halting and beginning to reverse the global incidence of malaria by 2015. The report shows—unquestionably—that this target has been achieved. Fifty-seven countries have reduced their malaria cases by 75 percent in line with the World Health Assembly's target for 2015" (WHO 2015: iv). According to the summary of the report: "The proportion of children infected with malaria parasites has halved in endemic areas of Africa since 2000. Infection prevalence among children aged 2–10 years is estimated to have declined from 33 percent in 2000 to 16 percent in 2015 (UI: 14–19 percent), with three-quarters of this change occurring after 2005" (WHO 2015: x).

The increase in the proportion of malaria cases in Keru and Tenga, the vast majority of which concerned children under ten years of age, does not mean, however, that the government's determination to fight malaria has failed. It could suggest that the focused interventions, including the frequent use of the rapid diagnostic tests (RDTs) and the availability of artemisinin-based combination therapy (ACT), had been a success. The WHO points out a number of reasons why countries like Burkina Faso have difficulty demonstrating a decline in malaria cases at the same speed as some other countries (WHO 2015: 40–53). For example, rates of decline in malaria incidence and mortality are slower in high-burden countries. Moreover, countries with weak health systems have difficulty providing malaria prevention interventions such as insecticide-treated mosquito nets (ITN) and indoor residual spraying (IRS), as well as providing intermittent preventive treatment (IPT) of pregnant women and infants during antenatal and postnatal care. Furthermore, since 2006, the health policy in Burkina Faso has encouraged health workers to use first-line malaria treatment presumptively for undiagnosed cases of fever. If health staff, during a clinical consultation, suspected a case of fever to be malaria, they were encouraged to label the disease as malaria and prescribe the relevant treatment. The RDT for malaria, in which a dipstick placed in a drop of blood from a finger prick checks for malaria antigens (Bonko et al. 2019), was introduced in 2006 as a simple alternative to microscopy. The RDT is very easy to use and provides health workers with evidence for their malaria diagnoses.[2]

The local health statistics in Keru and Tenga call, however, for some reflection. Does the disease pattern noted in the monthly reports actually reflect the overall disease pattern in these villages? Why did the proportion of malaria diagnoses increase over the years? These figures, I argue, are related to the relatively low use of public health facilities in this area.[3] In what follows, I discuss this pattern of disease diagnosis as an expression of what I call a "supply-demand nexus"—that is, rural citizens demanded those services they

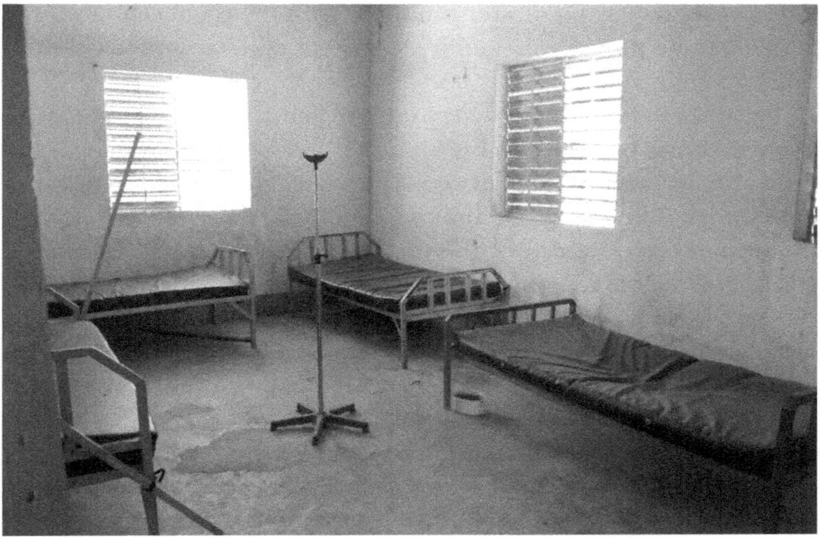

Figure 6.1. Admission room, rural dispensary, Burkina Faso (© Helle Samuelsen 2023)

knew could to be supplied. The patients and mothers of sick children knew that the health staff had the capacity to diagnose fever as malaria, and they knew from previous visits that such a diagnosis would be accompanied by a prescription for medicines that were likely to be in stock.

Diagnostic Repertoires

The rural dispensaries typically consist of a couple of buildings; one is reserved for general consultations and vaccinations while the other is used for deliveries and mother-child health care. The dispensary in Tenga had existed for many years and was already an established institution when I visited the village for the first time in 1996. The dispensary in Keru, however, was constructed some years later on the initiative of a successful "son of the village" who managed to mobilize a French NGO for its construction. The dispensary was sparsely furnished, with only a couple of cement benches and a few public health posters on the walls of the waiting room. The consultation room and rooms for admitted patients had an absolute minimum of equipment and instruments. The storage room held food supplements, and posters on the wall of the room explained the amount to be provided for undernourished children and women at risk.

The dispensary buildings were built of cement, in the style typical of government buildings in Burkina Faso. As most of the villages did not yet have electricity, solar panels had become increasingly common for providing light and for charging batteries. However, neither the dispensary in Keru nor the one in Tenga had stable electricity, even after the village was connected to the electrical grid in 2019. Instead, a gas refrigerator was used to keep the vaccines cold. The dispensaries did not have running water or modern sanitation facilities, but latrines had been constructed. Staff houses were located next to the dispensaries, and the health staff were posted at the specific facilities for two to four years before they were supposed to rotate to another post.[4] The fact that the staff lived next door meant that the villagers, in principle, had access to professional care 24/7 (unless the staff members were absent).

The dispensary in Keru was staffed with two government-trained nurses: *le major*[5] had overall responsibility, and *la matrone* was in charge of maternity and child health care, including vaccinations. The nurses had two years of training, while the third staff member, the assistant midwife (Agent Iténerant de Santé or AIS), who also helped with vaccination activities, had only one year of training. In addition, a village volunteer was responsible for the medical depot. On most days, the atmosphere at the dispensary was quiet, with only a few patients waiting for consultation during the morning hours. I passed by one morning in November 2013 with my local interpreter and Thomas, my main contact in the village. It was very tranquil; there were no admitted patients, and two women with their small children sat outside waiting to be called in. The nurse was in the consultation room finishing a consultation with a mother and her small boy, and his cries were the only sounds in the otherwise quiet building.

The dispensaries in Tenga and Keru were sparsely equipped. As Amadou, the nurse in charge at the dispensary in Keru, told me: "Our diagnostics are essentially based on the clinical signs, the physical signs, and simple examinations as for example the rapid diagnostic test. As we are not well equipped in terms of material and personnel, there are examinations that we cannot do."[6] The dearth of equipment clearly limited the health professionals' diagnostic repertoire. Because they had only a scale and the rapid diagnostic test, they mainly relied on their experience and their "clinical gaze" (Foucault 2012). For many years, the main focus of the primary health care system in Burkina Faso had been mother-child health and malaria (Ministère de la Santé 2011). This policy was expressed through prenatal screening of pregnant women, activities to encourage mothers to deliver at the health facilities, vaccination campaigns, and food supplement programs for vulnerable pregnant women and small children.

The dispensary staff are supposed to be the first health care contact for rural citizens. Some of the assigned nurses clearly felt that being responsible for the daily management of the dispensary was a heavy burden. "This is not always an easy task," Lankoandé, the new nurse in charge at the dispensary in Tenga, explained. "I just arrived after finishing my training for the CSPS [dispensary]. I only arrived last Sunday. I will say that there are many things here at the dispensary that I don't know about yet. After nursing school, I went to Ouahigouya at a Medical Center [Centre Medical]. This is the first time I work at a dispensary." Lankoandé had been through some training for the head nursing position, but he clearly found the task overwhelming. He had no previous experience working in a dispensary, and his two colleagues were also relatively new; the assistant nurse had been working at the facility for ten months, the birth attendant for four months. Furthermore, he explained that they faced language problems: "Here, people speak Bissa or Mooré, but I don't understand these languages well. Here, the women don't understand the French that we speak. One of my colleagues is Mossi, the other is Senoufo, and I am Gourmantché. Often, we do our best in Mooré, but if we don't succeed in understanding each other, we need an interpreter." Lankoandé's mother tongue was Gourmantché, and he was fluent in French, the administrative language in Burkina Faso, but, as he noted, most inhabitants in this area speak either Mooré or Bissa.

I encountered Lankoandé and his two colleagues at the Tenga dispensary deeply engaged in completing the monthly report, which had to be submitted the following day to the district health office. Lankoandé explained that they had to be meticulous when completing the report, which consisted of a series of tables,[7] as he had been assigned to this dispensary because the chief district medical officer had identified problems with the reports submitted by his predecessor (see also Samuelsen 2022).

The increase in malaria diagnoses is very clear if we look at the figures from Tenga in the table below where we have data from 2001, 2010, and 2013. In 2001, 28.4 percent of all patients at the dispensary in Tenga were diagnosed with uncomplicated malaria. In 2010, the diagnosis had increased to 35.4 percent of all patients and in 2013 to 46.4 percent. The figures from the dispensary in Keru show that more than 50 percent of its cases in January 2010 and 55.7 percent of cases in January 2013 were diagnosed with malaria.

The clinical encounter at the dispensaries followed a standard procedure: the patient (or mother with a sick child) entered the consultation room, where the nurse in charge was sitting behind a desk. The nurse asked a few questions about the condition and specific symptoms. In some cases, the nurse examined the patient (lifting the eyelids to look for anemia) or checked for fever with a thermometer, if available, or using their hands. After a short conversation and examination, the nurse would write a prescription and ask the patient to go to the medical depot to get the medicines (if injections were needed, this included needles and syringes, which were to be brought back to the nurse to be administered). The consultation process itself was routinized: the main component in the consultation was a short exchange between the patient or caregiver and the nurse with the purpose of diagnosing the illness and deciding on the treatment.

Table 6.1. Diagnoses of patients at CSPS Tenga and CSPS Keru (prepared by Helle Samuelsen based on monthly reports from dispensaries)

CSPS Tenga	Jan 2001	Jan 2001	Jan 2010	Jan 2010	Jan 2013	Jan 2013	CSPS K-eru	Jan 2010	Jan 2010	Jan 2013	Jan 2013
Uncomplicated malaria	28.4%	38	35.4%	177	46.4%	434		51.8%	195	55.7%	241
Complicated malaria	3.7%	5	3%	15	0.4%	4		4.3%	16	0.9%	4
Undetermined fever	0%	0	0%	0	0%	0		0%	0	0%	0
All cases		134		500		936			376		433

The diagnostic repertoire was thus quite small. The limited equipment, the strong focus on mother-child health care, and Burkina Faso's commitment to treating malaria together with the strategy of presumptive treatment for malaria contributed to the disease pattern reflected in the monthly reports, where malaria was the predominant diagnosis. Although the list of possible diagnoses provided on the monthly report form was fairly long, the actual diagnostic repertoire at the rural health dispensary was quite narrow.

Standards and Routines

For many years, opportunistic presumptive treatment (OPT) of fever was provided through primary health care facilities in many parts of Africa, including Burkina Faso. In order to avoid overdiagnosing fever as malaria, with the accompanying adverse effects for patients and skewed data for malaria control programs, the rapid diagnostic test was introduced as a simple, easy-to-distribute medical technology. The "factual" character of the test result—that is, are there malaria antigens or not—facilitated standardization of diagnosis, responded to the demand for "unbiased" counting (Adams 2016; Erikson 2016; Wendland 2016), and served as a signature of the state in the fragile context of rural health care. After the introduction of the RDT, health workers did not have to rely only on their clinical skills—that is, their ability to interpret symptoms—and they were not as dependent on the patient's history to make a diagnosis. If the patient reported fever, they would apply the test, and then, based on the test result, they prescribed medicines.

The health care workers I met at the rural dispensaries all emphasized malaria as the main health problem in the communities they served. Lankoandé said, "Here, the most serious problem is malaria, which is devastating." The district medical officer explained, "We still have some work to do. We have the rapid diagnostic test, but that does not give us permission to make irrational analyses. We have said that we do the RDT in relation to all fever cases, and in cases where there was fever during the previous seventy-two hours. But not all cases of fever are necessarily malaria."[8] Later in our conversation, he suggested that the dispensaries perhaps performed too many tests. However, from the perspective of the health workers, the introduction of the RDT confirmed that the fight against malaria continued to be the main health priority, and it provided them with a tangible technology that both expanded their diagnostic repertoire and strengthened their diagnostic authority (Pare Toe and Samuelsen 2020). Eleanor Hutchinson and colleagues identified the same boost in legitimacy among drugstore owners in Tanzania during a trial in which the rapid diagnostic test was introduced (Hutchinson, Chandler et al. 2015; Hutchinson, Reyburn et al. 2017). The patients, for their part, also welcomed the RDT, as it provided them with a unique and professional answer to their health problem as well as a solution in the form of a prescription.

While the WHO's ICD provided a standardization of disease categories and a common diagnostic language for health care professionals around the world, the OPT and RDT standardized diagnostic procedures in Burkina Faso, filled a gap in a health system that previously had neither the equipment nor the human capacity to arrive at a scientifically based diagnosis. Standards create homogeneity and facilitate global coordination (Brunsson and Jacobsson 2000: 1). Standardization is defined, according to Stefan Timmermans and Steven Epstein, as a "process of constructing uniformities across time and space through the generation of agreed-upon rules" (2010: 71). There are, of course, also standards for defining a standard itself. The International Organization for Standardization defines a standard as "a document established by consensus and approved by a recognized body, that provides, for common and repeated use, rules, guidelines or characteristics for activities or their results aimed at the achievement of the optimum degree of order in a given context" (Brunsson and Jacobsson 2000: 15).

Having standards is usually seen as praiseworthy; one aspires to live up to them. Standardization, on the other hand, is often derogatory in its popular usage. Although standards are often formulated by experts, they may come to function as an alternative to expert knowledge (Timmermans and Epstein 2010: 71). The licensed health care workers were instructed in how to use the standard procedures (e.g., the rapid diagnostic test) and how to report the diagnoses in standardized ways. These uniform procedures contributed to ensuring homogeneity in health care reporting across the different health facilities and across time. The fact that the RDT was almost the only medical technology available at the rural dispensaries may suggest that most fevers were diagnosed as malaria, as the health care pro-

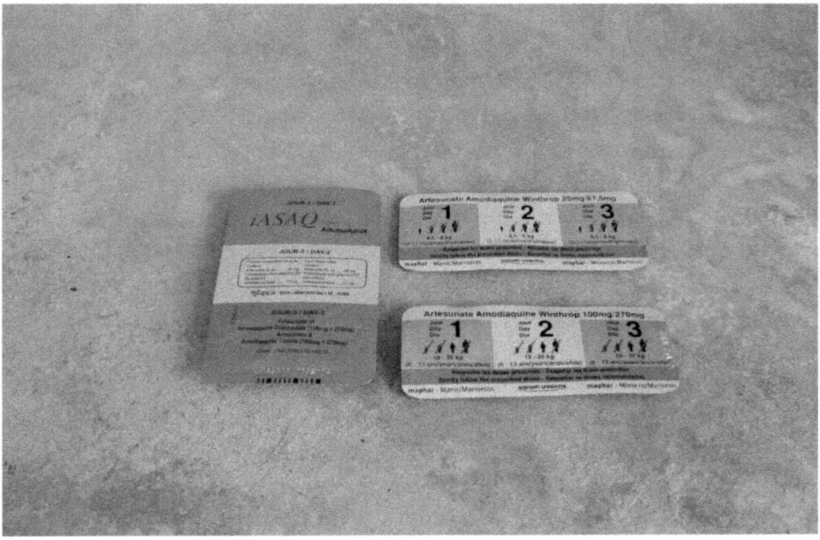

Figure 6.2. Malaria medicine, Burkina Faso (© Helle Samuelsen 2023)

fessionals did not have the expertise or diagnostic equipment to arrive at other accurate, evidence-based diagnoses for fever.

The routine consultation process described above, combined with the standardized diagnostic procedures, made the outcome of a visit to the dispensary rather predictable for patients. The citizens of Tenga and Keru had some certainty in knowing what was offered at the clinic, particularly in cases of fever: a quick conversation, a fingertip prick, and a prescription that could be "cashed" at the medical depot. As we shall see in the following case, even when the RDT showed a negative result, patients were often prescribed antimalarial treatment and the cases were thus registered as malaria.

Fever

Malaria

Thirty-five-year-old Alimata, one of my interlocutors in Keru, lived alone with her three children, who were seven years, five years, and ten months of age. Her husband, Idrissa, was working on a plantation in Côte d'Ivoire, sending money home to her once a year. Her youngest child had been ill with *palu*—short for *paludisme*, the

French word for malaria—for three days. He suffered from *corps chaud* (warm body) and was coughing. Alimata used the local term *yinwingre* for malaria. Alimata spoke in short sentences when she explained the various treatment options she had tried. First, she went to the local market to buy some herbs, which she had boiled and given the child to drink every morning for three days. On the second day, she had also taken him to the dispensary, as his body was still warm. There, they tested for malaria, which, according to Alimata, showed a negative result. However, the nurse prescribed artesunate-amodiaquine as well as paracetamol and some cough medicine; the child was also given one injection at the consultation. Alimata paid 1,500 CFA [franc] (US$3.00) for the medicines. Because of the treatment, the child was categorized in the statistics as having malaria, although the RDT test result was negative.[9]

Alimata's case was in many ways typical. As discussed in previous chapters, the choice of whom to consult in case of sickness is ambiguous. In Keru, mothers of sick children often tried various indigenous treatments at home first. If the symptoms persisted, they would eventually go to the dispensary where they knew that their children, in case of fever, would receive a prescription for malaria treatment. As Alimata explained, "I only go to the dispensary if the disease does not finish [with home treatment], if it is grave, because I don't have money. My husband is in Côte d'Ivoire, he only rarely sends me 5,000 CFA [franc] [US$8.50]." Alimata's child was diagnosed as suffering from malaria despite the negative test result, and Alimata was aware of that. Data from other studies in Burkina confirm this practice. Zeno Bisoffi and colleagues (2009) found that around 80 to 85 percent of patients with a negative malaria test were nevertheless treated for malaria. The female volunteer in charge of the medical depot attached to the dispensary confirmed that *palu* was the most common disease. The ACT malaria treatment included a three-day course in which adults were to take two tablets twice a day while children were to take one tablet per day. A packet of malaria medicine for children was sold for 100 CFA [franc] (US$0.16), and a course of treatment for adults was sold for 300 CFA [franc] (as of 2015).

When going through the notes of my interviews with mothers in Keru and Tenga, I saw a similar tendency: mothers consulted the dispensary in cases of "warm body" to a somewhat greater extent than they did for other illnesses, although they rarely articulated this preference explicitly. However, Adissa, a Bissa woman interviewed in 2010, did speak of it. She explained that she took her children to the dispensary "par-ce-que le corps chaud se soigne a l'hospital" (because warm body is treated at the hospital). Mariam, a young Mossi woman who for many years lived in Côte d'Ivoire and in Ouagadougou, said that the two most common diseases of her eight-month-old child were *palu* and *pugnondre* (stomach problems). The *palu* is caused by mosquitoes, she said, while *pugnondre* is related to the "sortie de la lune" (position of the moon). She consulted the dispensary for *palu*, while traditional medicine worked better in cases of *pugnondre*.

Fever was the symptom mentioned most often by women when talking about their children's recent illnesses and when talking about the frequency of illnesses more generally. In a semistructured questionnaire conducted with fifty women in Keru in 2010, fever was the most commonly mentioned illness, and many women said that in the most recent episode of child fever, they had consulted the dispensary. It is my impression that use of the dispensary had increased over the years compared to self-medication and to consultations with traditional healers. In the most recent demographic health survey (INSD 2021), 22 percent of children under five years of age had suffered from fever within the previous two weeks, and among them 75 percent had consulted biomedical health services.[10] A few women expressed a strong skepticism toward traditional medicine, though many others explained that their first action in case of illness was to use various types of herbal medicines at home, either based on advice from an elderly woman in the compound or after having consulted a traditional healer in the village. A few of the women who preferred to go straight to the dispensary told me that it took a lot of time to use herbal treatments, as one had to go to the bush first to collect the necessary bark, leaves, or roots. Others argued that their preference for herbal medicine was based on the high cost of medicines at the dispensary. Though I am not able to substantiate this statistically, it is my impression that women whose husbands had migrated to another country were more inclined to use herbal medicine because of its lower cost, as remittances were meager or arrived at irregular intervals.

Mothers of sick children did not complain if they were not given exact information about their child's diagnosis. Instead, they were more concerned about "doing away" (Mol 2002) with the symptoms by getting a prescription. As in Hanne Mogensen's (2005) study of rural clinics in Uganda, the little piece of paper with the written prescription became a "token." The mothers sought to take pragmatic action in response to disease. Often their children had been ill for days before they decided to go to the dispensary, and often the mothers had tried other strategies before contacting the public health care facilities. They tried to be hopeful—and they looked for certainty. In a sense, they did find certainty at the dispensary: parents knew that their children would be examined and given some medicine, and their experiential knowledge told them that this would happen in cases of fever. This is what I call the availability logic or the supply-demand nexus: sick people went to the public health services primarily with afflictions for which they knew treatment would be supplied. The standardized diagnostic procedure and treatment of fever was a way for both health professionals to care for the sick and for mothers to care for their children.

Invisible Illnesses

The health policies of Burkina Faso have, as mentioned, prioritized the availability of health facilities in rural areas, yet there are a number of factors that shape whether those facilities are used. Whether people have the possibility of traveling to a health facility also influences how likely they are to use it (Fainzang 1986; Haddad, Nougtara, and Fournier 2006; Samuelsen 2004b). Visiting a health facility can be expensive in terms of direct costs, such as payment for medicine and equipment, and indirect costs, such as lost working time. Furthermore, the quality of the patient-provider relationship affects utilization rates (Gilson, Palmer, and Schneider 2005; Samuelsen, Tersbol, and Mbuyita 2013; see also Kruk, Kujawski et al. 2018).

Rural citizens mainly consulted the primary health care facilities with cases of sickness corresponding to the limited repertoire of diseases the dispensaries were able to diagnose and treat. Although fever was extremely common in Tenga and Keru, the monthly reports are remarkable for how few of the other diagnostic categories were actually used. Both anemia and malnutrition were visible in these communities, and the dispensaries distributed daily food supplements to the mothers of malnourished children (aged six to fifty-nine months). However, these two diagnoses were rarely mentioned in the monthly reports. Other illnesses, such as sexually transmitted diseases, mental illness, and dental problems, were nearly absent from the monthly reports. When asked why the rate at which malaria was diagnosed was increasing in Burkina while decreasing in other African countries, the regional director of health explained:

> Perhaps they have managed to do more scientific studies, perhaps it is also a question about the diagnostic tools used, and apart from that they have more options for diagnosing in laboratories, whereas here, until recently, we have relied on the clinical suspicion only. Thus, the comparison is a bit complicated. Another explanation is that we also have a fight at the community level, where we do not perform well. We distribute one mosquito net for two persons where other places each person gets a mosquito net, and you know that people do not necessarily sleep in pairs of two. I know that in many countries both the diagnostics and the treatment are done better at the community level. We also have this strategy, but the funding has not been good, and if the funding is not there, it won't work. In my opinion, this is what explains the difference with other countries.

He argued that the high rate of malaria diagnosis in Burkina Faso might be due to health care workers relying on clinical suspicion (the clinical gaze) because they lacked proper laboratories. The country was also unable to provide an adequate number of mosquito nets or to establish good diagnostic facilities. While this is true, the high rates of malaria diagnosis could also be an unintended result of the widespread use of the rapid diagnostic test.

The monthly reports were sent to the chief medical officer of the district, where the data were entered into a database, providing district and regional management a far better overview of disease patterns.[11] The reports from the dispensaries have the best data available on morbidity and mortality in rural parts of the country (excepting the data generated from the demographic health survey, which is conducted at intervals of five to ten years).

In this chapter, I have noted that the proportion of cases diagnosed as malaria was relatively high and apparently increased over time. I am interested in what this could tell us about the relationship between rural citizens and the state—or, more specifically, about the relationship between rural citizens and the public health care system. What kind of services did rural citizens expect from public health facilities, and how did this demand match the supplies provided by the government? Zooming in on the relationship between rural citizens and the health care system allows us to see how the social contract between the government and villagers played out in everyday life. The term "public health," Ruth Prince and Rebecca Marsland (2014) discuss, refers to the duties of the modern state to protect and care for the health of its citizens.

The citizens of Keru—in my experience—rarely criticized the health system openly when medicine was out of stock or when personnel were absent. They did not claim their entitlements as citizens with rights to public health care (Petryna 2002, 2013b); rather, they shared an ontology of marginality. In the consultation room, the patients conformed themselves to a legitimate order, to use Weber's terminology, where the health worker represented governmental authority (Weber 1978: 31). However, as in the case of Caro, described in chapter 2, they often felt uncomfortable in these relationships. Rural citizens were thus left with unsolved illnesses that the public health care system was unprepared to recognize or act on.

Another related question is, of course, why so few were diagnosed with sexually transmitted diseases, heart problems, high blood pressure, or diabetes. Also, why were there almost no mental health concerns—and no dental problems at all? In other words, a huge number of illnesses and conditions became invisible since only a small fraction of them were brought forward to the public health care system. I suggest that we look at this supply-demand nexus as a "technology of invisibility," similar to that described by Joao Biehl (2005) in his analysis of the nonregistered AIDS deaths of marginal groups in Bahia, Brazil.

Statistics are collected at the primary level of the health care system, in this case from the dispensary, and fed into the bureaucracy, informing not only national policies but eventually also international policies and guidelines, including those promulgated by the WHO. Statistics play a crucial role for politicians and policy-makers. According to Morten Jerven, "Poor numbers fundamentally shape what we know about development in sub-Saharan Africa, which in turn shapes how decisions are made" (Jerven 2013:4). Statistical indicators are, as Sally E. Merry says, "fundamental to modern forms of governmentality" (Merry 2011: S83). The demand for metrics and the increased need for systems of quantification have been widely discussed in political anthropology and beyond (Foucault 2012; Jerven 2008; Porter 1996; Scott 1998).

Labeling all fever cases as *paludisme simple*, whether that happened because of the government policy of treating undiagnosed cases of fever as malaria or because it was the habituated practice of health workers (or some combination of both), confirmed to the public and to policy-makers that malaria was the main health problem in rural Burkina Faso. Whether all these patients really suffered from malaria is, of course, unknown. But we know from conversations with the inhabitants of Tenga and Keru that they also suffered from a range of illnesses other than fever. The brief, routinized consultations and the limited diagnostic repertoire contributed to the exclusion of diseases other than malaria from the monthly reports and the public health care statistics. As the monthly reports focused increasingly on malaria, other diseases became invisible.

Ambiguous Relationships

The relationship between the government's health representatives at the village level and rural citizens appeared to be fragile. In this chapter, I have pointed to the fragile situation that arose when the limited diagnostic repertoire of the dispensary and the subsequent underutilization of the primary health care facility left rural citizens without much support from government services. Furthermore, the monthly reports led policy-makers to focus narrowly on malaria treatment, not taking into account the increasing burden of other communicable as well as noncommunicable diseases.

Caro, Thomas's daughter, provides another example of the fragile relationship between the government and villagers. As a teenager, Caro suffered for a number of years from an eye infection, and the sight in one of her eyes was seriously affected. Every time I asked her about it, she assured me that she was taking medicine and that it was improving, but the strong sunlight clearly disturbed her, and she tried to stay in the shade as much as possible. After several conversations about her eye infection, I finally persuaded her to let me take her to the eye hospital in Zorgo, a town located more than a hundred kilometers from her village. She was reluctant, but she was encouraged by her parents. Thomas, her father, went with us, as he wanted to be checked for his increasingly annoying cataract. After a short wait, she was called in for consultation. The doctor, a fairly young eye specialist, asked her to sit in a chair in order to be examined. She hardly responded to his questions, and it became clear that she had actually visited the hospital before. The doctor scolded her, as he could see that she had stopped taking the medicines he had previously prescribed and that her cornea was damaged. While she had not lost sight in the infected eye, the damage was permanent, and the doctor strongly advised her to follow the treatment in order to save her eye.

Such a reluctant relationship with the public health facility reveals the complexity of bio-citizenship. Caro's evasive and ambivalent use of the public health facility in relation to her eye infection and to the delivery of her son, as described in the introduction, was not unique. She did not claim her entitlements as a bio-citizen of Burkina Faso with a right to be assisted in delivering her child. Although the dispensary was available and to a certain extent also accessible, Caro, like many other rural citizens, only used the services sporadically. Accessibility continued to be an issue, not least for women, who often needed to ask permission or at least ask for money from their husbands. Transport, too, was a real problem for many people, even though it had been a long-term ambition to reduce the distance to the nearest health facility for both urban and rural residents.

Metrics and Politics

While it certainly is advantageous that a common global system of disease classification exists (namely, the ICD), and while it is useful that first-line health care facilities systematically report their activities and that the reporting data are compiled and analyzed, it is still relevant to ask critical questions about the knowledge produced by these universal standards and reports. Vincanne Adams explains that "metrics are technologies of counting, but specifically technologies of counting that form global knowledge. Metrics used today are imagined to offer uniform and standardized conversations about how best to intervene, how best to conceptualize health and disease, how best to both count and be accountable, and how best to pay for it all" (Adams 2016: 6). The knowledge produced by the monthly reports from the Keru and Tenga dispensaries informed us of a heavy and increasing malaria burden in this particular area; this knowledge continues to shape the overall health care priorities of the country.

What does this knowledge reveal and conceal? According to my analysis, the data and this type of reporting reveal a strong government commitment to fight malaria, with a particular focus on mothers and children, while also acknowledging the limited diagnostic capacity at rural health care facilities. However, this data production also reveals another aspect not yet discussed extensively in the anthropological literature: namely, rural citizens navigate the system according to their experiences with the services provided at the dispensaries. When they see that the nurses at the rural dispensaries are able to act on cases of fever, use the rapid diagnostic test, and prescribe available medicine, patients tend to use the facilities in exactly such instances. If most fevers are diagnosed as malaria and many other symptoms are treated at home or by local specialists, the government's policy of focusing on malaria does not reflect the actual disease pattern of the country. The system of monthly reporting and the routinized practices at health facilities in which the RDT is the most important diagnostic technology produce metrics indicating that Burkina Faso, contrary to many other countries in Africa (WHO 2015), is experiencing a heavy and increasing malaria burden.

The regional director of health services, Dr. Sawadogo, was well aware that Burkina Faso was experiencing an epidemiological transition where so-called noncommunicable diseases were becoming more widespread alongside a continuing high level of infectious diseases, a development that poses a challenge for the health care system. At an interview in 2015, he said, "The last surveys show that we are in an epidemiological transition, or an additional epidemiology on top of the old diseases. In 2013, we had a national survey on chronic and noncommunicable diseases, which showed that almost 23 percent of adults in our area suffer from hypertension." He pointed to the lack of government funding for the health care sector in general:

> The actual problems are related to our finances. This includes different aspects: the demand for health care is increasing, but the number of health staff does not match the demand. Also, our budget for repairs and improvements of our equipment and infrastructure is limited, and the logistics of our vehicles for supervision and motorcycles for vaccinations

> are part of our financial challenges. We are also in a phase of decentralization involving a transfer of resources and power to the municipalities, but the capacity of the ministry to advise the municipalities is very slow. . . . Over the years, you see a change in the new generation [of health staff]. There is an expression saying "little money—little work." You sense that more and more.

Thus, according to Dr. Sawadogo, they did not have enough personnel, the equipment and infrastructure were poor, and they furthermore struggled with decentralization, where both resources and power were transferred to local councils. The regional director of health was clearly frustrated, as he felt that the regions had neither the capacity nor the power to live up to the aims and indicators stipulated in the national health policy.

Conclusion

By exploring the diagnostic routines at the dispensaries and following individual cases of illness, we discovered the various ways in which the social contract between the government's health care services and rural citizens played out in everyday life. The duties of the modern state to protect and care for the health of its citizens, as embedded in the term "public health," were not fulfilled. Burkina Faso is a poor country with an underfinanced health care system. Both the regional director of health services and the district medical officer were enthusiastic about their data portal, where they have access to the latest health care data. That is, of course, encouraging. But, as I hope to have demonstrated in this chapter, there is a need to look critically at the metrics—and the critical scrutiny of health data must, I think, start at the village dispensary. While the data reveal a strong focus on malaria and identify specific characteristics of the population's health, the data are not necessarily accurate, and they conceal other important information about health, disease, and health care-seeking practices.

Notes

1. International Classification of Diseases (ICD).
2. The rapid diagnostic test used in Burkina Faso is based on *Plasmodium falciparum* histidine-rich protein-2 (PfHRP2). *P. falciparum* is the most common malaria parasite in Burkina Faso (Bonko et al. 2019).

3. See chapter 5.
4. Occasionally, nurses may stay for a longer period, particularly if they have their family with them.
5. *Infirmier-chef de poste* (ICP) is the head nurse of the dispensary.
6. Interview conducted in November 2015.
7. The diagnostic system has changed a couple of times since I first looked at the monthly reports back in 1996–1997.
8. Interview conducted in 2015.
9. According to the official policy, malaria treatment should only be prescribed if the RDT is positive (Ministère de la Santé 2017).
10. In the DHS survey, this includes public, private, and NGO biomedical health facilities as well as pharmacies and itinerant medicine providers (Institut National de la Statistique et de la Démographie 2021: 35).
11. I do not know exactly when this district introduced the database.

Chapter 7
Moments of State Presence

COVID-19: A Global Disruption

The COVID-19 pandemic affected most people across the globe in one way or another. During the two-year period from 2020 to 2022, more than 578 million people tested positive for COVID-19, more than six million people died, around four billion people were vaccinated, and the vast majority of the world's population experienced restrictions on their mobility or various types of hygienic injunctions.[1] The COVID-19 pathogen traveled incredibly quickly and took the whole world by surprise, although warnings about emerging epidemics with the potential to evolve into pandemics had been articulated (Lakoff 2017; WEF 2016; WHO 2018). A number of researchers and organizations had already voiced concern that global flows of people and goods, climate change, and hotspots with favorable conditions for animal-to-human disease transmission created the risk of new pandemics (Brown and Kelly 2014). The COVID-19 pandemic has demonstrated the importance of studying uncertainties, risks, emergencies, and crises from an anthropological perspective (Caduff 2015; Chigudu 2019; Ecks 2020; Erikson 2018; Hewlett and Hewlett 2008; Kelly, Keck, and Lynteris 2019; Lakoff 2017; Lynteris 2014; Lynteris and Poleykett 2018; Manderson, Burke, and Wahlberg 2021; Mason 2016; Team and Manderson 2020; Whyte 2014).

Furthermore, the course of the pandemic showed that few countries were sufficiently prepared for such a fast-moving contagious pathogen, which spread to more than two hundred countries and closed down societies for months (Kandel et al. 2020). The fragility of globalization with its accelerated interconnectedness was suddenly exposed, and in contrast to other recent epidemics, which had touched mainly the Global South, cases of COVID-19 were identified across the globe. In addition to the direct consequences—including death, sickness, massive test systems, the development of new vaccines, and the implementation of huge vaccination programs—the pandemic had marked and long-lasting impacts on people's livelihoods, financial well-being, and access to health care services, even after the end of the global lockdown, particularly in low-income societies like Burkina Faso (Team and Manderson 2020). Studies show that COVID-19 has intensified precarity and contributed to further exclusion and marginalization of people who already live precarious lives and who already struggle to access public services (Bjertrup 2021; Adama Diallo et al. 2022; Gamlin et al. 2021; MacGregor et al. 2022; Team and Manderson 2020).

In early 2020, the virus compelled governments around the world to formulate preparedness and response plans and to introduce a range of precautionary measures, many of which had serious implications for everyday life as well as for local and global economies. The introduction of severe measures such as enforcing nightly curfews, closing borders, quarantining towns with cases of infection, closing down schools and marketplaces, and requiring face masks raises questions about how citizens responded to such disruptions. The government of Burkina Faso developed a response plan at a very early stage of the epidemic that to a large extent mirrored the vertical, state-led lockdown models adopted in Europe and Asia with advice from WHO (MacGregor et al. 2022). In this final chapter, I shift attention from the everyday routines of the dispensary in Keru to changes in state–citizen dynamics in Burkina Faso during the COVID-19 pandemic from 2020 to 2022.[2]

In previous chapters, I have argued that although the state was present at the village level in the form of schools, dispensaries, and municipal offices, it was also absent as equipment, staff, and diagnostic capacities at these facilities were limited. The previous chapters also demonstrate that everyday life for most citizens of Keru was lived without much contact with state representatives, although the "desire" for the state and its services was present (Street 2014: 21–23). However, during COVID-19, the state took on a much more visible role when formulating plans to contain and prevent the epidemic and when enforcing restrictive measures. The state, government, and president were no longer "absent imaginaries" but rather institutions and representatives who made decisions and enforced measures—virtually overnight—that unsettled the everyday life of citizens in concrete ways. In this chapter, I zoom in on how both the government and ordinary citizens responded to the pandemic and examine how local responses to the epidemic and the precautionary measures introduced by the government affected and (temporarily) changed the relationship between citizens and the state.

At first, in the early phase of the pandemic, many people expressed ambiguity and skepticism about the danger of COVID-19 in Burkina Faso, where people have lived through many epidemics. Particularly in the larger cities, there were sizable protests against the border closures and market lockdowns, as these measures dramatically affected the day-to-day economy of ordinary people. Later, despite the pandemic's relatively mild course in Burkina Faso with only registered 366 deaths and 20,599 confirmed cases (as of 26 January 2022), COVID-19 continued to be talked about as an exceptional disease, as an epidemic like no previous epidemics. I argue here that the exceptionality of COVID-19 was not so much related to its specific risks or symptoms, but rather to the fact that people had never before experienced a government that introduced such severe general restrictions in order to safeguard the health of the population. The otherwise "absent" or distant government had suddenly stepped in and deployed its sovereign authority and biopower to "discipline the population" to pre-empt an uncertain future. Momentarily, the state demonstrated its wish to care for its citizens, a gesture that in itself was recognized by many.

History of Epidemics in Burkina Faso

Many citizens who took part in our COVID-19 study in Bobo-Dioulasso emphasized that epidemics have always been part of everyday life in Burkina Faso. Malaria, which continues to be endemic throughout the country, is but one of several epidemics profoundly impacting life (and death) in the country. Smallpox was well-known in West Africa before colonization and spread to the Americas with the slave trade.[3] As mentioned in chapter 4, Cotton Mather, a prominent American in the early eighteenth century, learned about the inoculation technique from an enslaved person given to him by his constituency in 1706. Onesimus, as Mather had named him, had been inoculated as a child in what is now Burkina Faso, where he had obtained immunity after a mild case of the disease (Watts 1997: 113). The inoculation technique, in which material from a smallpox scab is rubbed into a small cut in the skin, was used in West Africa to contain and control the disease. In his book on the history of epidemics, Watts argues, however, that smallpox most probably was not transmitted by an enslaved person, but by one of the Europeans who worked on the slave ships (Watts 1997: 110).[4]

Smallpox incidence in West Africa followed a seasonal pattern with peaks in the dry months (March and April), but due to a lack of surveillance systems and underreporting, the actual number of cases and related deaths is not known (Foege, Millar, and Henderson 1975). An eradication program was launched in Burkina Faso (then called Upper Volta) in 1966 with support from WHO and USAID with the aim of vaccinating the entire population within three years. From 1967 to 1972, more than eight million people in Upper Volta were vaccinated, and it is estimated that more than 80 percent of the people in most age groups were reached. During the same period, about 28 million children in West Africa were vaccinated against measles (Foege, Millar, and Henderson 1975). Overall, the smallpox eradication program was seen as a huge success, and it impelled the global health community, including WHO, to launch other eradication programs.

Epidemic outbreaks of yellow fever occurred a number of times in West Africa, but with very few registered cases in Burkina Faso. Again, it is difficult to get exact data on the actual number of cases. This is mainly because the symptoms of yellow fever resemble those of a number of other tropical diseases, laboratory capacity in the country was insufficient, and there was what Dr. Rubert Boyce in 1911 termed notification fear, a tendency to underreport the actual number of deaths for political or commercial reasons (Watts 1997: 218). River blindness (onchocerciasis), a disease caused by a parasitic worm spread by the blackfly, was endemic in Burkina Faso, particularly among people living in the river valleys. After a severe drought from 1968 to 1974, the Onchocerciasis Control Program (OCP) was launched, led by WHO.[5] At that time, malaria, schistosomiasis, trypanosomiasis (sleeping sickness), and river blindness were all endemic in this region. The early program aimed to control the blackfly vector by repeated spraying of infected river basins with degradable insecticides. After 1982, when ivermectin was discovered, the control strategy shifted to free distribution of ivermectin through the public health system (McMillan 1995: 1–8). As a disease control program with large donor investments, the OCP was a success. However, as McMillan concluded, while the program may have provided new agricultural potential in the river basins, there were still many problems to address in order to significantly improve people's living conditions (McMillan 1995: 136).

Several cholera outbreaks have also been registered in Burkina Faso, and, as with most other epidemics, it mostly affected the poor. Cholera was first noted in Africa in 1836, with only a few outbreaks between then and the 1970s (Mengel et al. 2014). The first registered cases of cholera were reported in Burkina Faso in 1971. Since then, the country has experienced five outbreaks, the latest of which was in 2005 (Kaboré et al. 2018).[6] Most epidemic control programs have been donor-driven, and WHO has played an essential role in technical design and political and economic support for these programs. In his historical overview of cholera epidemics in Africa, Myron Echenberg notes that "the WHO position on cholera in developing societies has often been paternalistic" with a tendency to alternately blame the Africans and apologize for them (Echenberg 2011: 178).

Measles and meningitis epidemics have also taken their toll on child health. Clinically diagnosed cases of measles have been documented by the Ministry of Health in Burkina Faso since 1984. The largest measles outbreak in Burkina Faso occurred in 1996 with minor outbreaks almost every year from 1997 to 2005 (Maradze, Nyoni, and Nyoni 2021). Because the child vaccination rate is high in Burkina Faso, the number of measles cases is much lower than it might otherwise be.[7] Burkina Faso is located within what is called the meningitis belt, which runs across the African continent from Senegal to Ethiopia. Before the mass vaccination campaign in 2010 with a new effective vaccine, outbreaks of meningitis were common during the Harmattan (the dry season, typically taking place from November through March). Today, the vaccine is part of the routine child vaccination program (Soeters et al. 2019).

As we shall see below, experiences from the AIDS epidemic are sometimes used to reflect broadly on COVID-19. The AIDS epidemic hit hard in Burkina Faso, although prevalence rates were much lower than in many countries in East Africa and Southern Africa.[8] The pandemic stretched over many years, from the early 1980s to today, causing great suffering for patients and their families. Stigma and difficulty accessing care and treatment continue to be a problem, particularly for people with few resources and fragile family relationships (Benton, Sangaramoorthy, and Kalofonos 2017; Dilger and Luig 2010; Gausset et al. 2012; Nguyen 2010; Samuelsen, Norgaard, and Ostergaard 2012; Whyte 2014). The World Bank estimates that 0.7 percent of the adult population between fifteen and forty-nine years of age in Burkina Faso were living with an HIV diagnosis in 2020.[9] While Ebola did not reach Burkina Faso, it was much feared and frequently discussed; for a period, borders between Burkina Faso and neighboring countries were closed in order to contain the epidemic and avoid transmission into the country.

This brief history of epidemics in Burkina Faso shows that the country has a lot of prior experience, and it was clear in the many conversations about COVID-19 that people drew on these prior experiences as they analyzed COVID-19. COVID-19 was seen as exceptional not only because it was a global pandemic rather than a local or regional epidemic and not only because the virus's rapid global spread began in China, but also because the measures taken to prevent and control the pandemic in Burkina were exceptional. I examine this in more detail in the section below.

Early Responses

The first case of COVID-19 in Burkina Faso was announced by the Ministry of Health on 9 March 2020 in a press briefing. Upon their return to Burkina Faso from a large religious congregation in Mulhouse, France, a priest and his wife tested positive. In the beginning, it took a few days to confirm results, as the samples had to be sent to Institut Pasteur in Senegal for analysis until the National Reference Laboratory for Influenza was upgraded to perform the PCR (polymerase chain reaction) tests for COVID-19. The first two cases created headlines in the news as well as on social media. The government promptly declared COVID-19 "a public health emergency,"[10] and a number of measures were introduced to prevent the virus from spreading. On 18 March, only nine days after the first identified cases in Burkina Faso, schools and universities were closed. Two days later, on 20 March, the president of Burkina Faso closed the borders and announced a curfew from 7:00 p.m. to 5:00 a.m., a ban on gatherings of more than fifty people, and the closure of restaurants and entertainment venues. Attending services in churches and mosques was banned, and on 26 March the government quarantined all cities that had declared COVID cases.[11]

By 5 April, 302 cases had been confirmed and forty-one patients had died (Besarabic 2020).[12] Based on the epidemiological development of the pandemic and the growing number of cases in Burkina Faso, the Ministry of Health developed a response plan (Plan de Preparation et de Riposte a l'Epidemie COVID-19 au Burkina Faso). The plan was published in March 2020[13] and included a thorough analysis of the country's current capacities and challenges related to prevention, diagnosis, and control of COVID-19. It emphasized that a large-scale outbreak was to be expected if effective interventions were not introduced (Ministère de la Santé 2020: 3). A national committee for the management of the COVID-19 epidemic was formed under the prime minister, and similar committees were established at regional and provincial levels. In addition, a group of medical and financial experts was engaged to supervise the implementation of the activities. The government of Burkina Faso had already reinforced its epidemic surveillance system after the West African Ebola epidemic in 2014–16. The Ministry of Health introduced a weekly epidemic survey form for each of the 1,896 dispensaries in the country to complete in order to provide the ministry with up-to-date information on potential outbreaks (Rasmussen 2017; Rasmussen and Sahay 2022). The form (Telegramme Lettre Officiel Hebdomaire) included a list of about fifteen potential epidemic diseases for which health staff should immediately report cases.[14]

During the early months of the epidemic, many people expressed uncertainty about how contagious the virus would be on the African continent. Kotim, a forty-five-year-old woman selling vegetables at the big market in Bobo-Dioulasso, expressed her doubts about the actual existence of the virus in Burkina Faso during a conversation in early May 2020:

> *Kotim:* First of all, in the morning you have to go to the market to sell your products. If you manage to get some money, you buy some condiments with that in the evening. But, if they tell you to go home and sit for a month, and you have children, how do you manage? Is that good? They

say that the disease returned here,[15] but I have not seen anyone who was identified with this disease. In any case, they say that it has returned. But I cannot say that I have seen such a disease. They say it has returned, we look, but we have not seen the disease.

Estelle: When it is said that the disease is here, but you say that you have not yet seen anybody with this disease, does that mean that you think that the disease does not exist?

Kotim: Exactly. According to me, the disease does not exist.

Estelle: But then, according to you, why does the government say the disease exists?

Kotim: The fact that it is our government who said that the disease exists, we follow it. If someone is in front of you, what they say is what you do. Otherwise, we have not seen the disease. We have heard about it. But we have not seen it. Since they are our leaders, if they say that the disease is there, it is there. That's why we follow him [the president]. If he says to wash our hands, we wash; if he says to close our noses, we close. If someone is in front of you, what they say to do is what you do. That's why. Otherwise, we have not seen the disease; we have only heard about it.

Estelle: According to you, the disease does not exist?

Kotim: According to me, the disease does not exist. Even if it exists, it does not exist in our country, in my opinion. (Interview, 6 May 2020)

Many people expressed their doubts about the existence of COVID-19 in Burkina Faso during the early months of the epidemic. This ambiguousness was, as Kotim remarked, related to the fact that nobody at that point had seen a case of COVID-19 within their families, in their neighborhood, or even on television (see also Samuelsen and Toé 2021). The disease's invisibility was mentioned by many of our interlocutors; they found it puzzling that the government talked a lot about the pandemic, but the authorities had not demonstrated the presence of the disease by showing a single case on television. Soungalo, who worked in a wholesale company, recognized COVID-19 as an actual disease, but, according to him, COVID-19 was just another kind of malaria:

In my opinion, I would say that it is a disease that cannot wipe out an African. Why? Because since birth, we have received injections against these types of diseases. In addition, I would think that there is not an African who had never suffered from malaria, cold, cough, or a fever. Thus, we are habituated to these kinds of diseases. But among the whites, they

> do not do the injections that we do here. Suppose a white baby who had not received the injections that we do here in young age. . . . Honestly, what the whites go through with many deaths due to this disease. If it was among us here, we would have had many more deaths than what the whites experience. (Interview, 6 May 2020)

While Soungalo talked about a certain robustness among the African population due to experiences with malaria, he also referenced the less robust health care system in the Global South, which would be less equipped to take care of many seriously ill patients.

Even though the Ministry of Health had started to announce the number of newly diagnosed COVID-19 cases and COVID-19 related deaths through daily press releases, many people continued to question the existence of the disease in Burkina Faso. Martin, a thirty-six-year-old bar manager, shared his thoughts about the likelihood of a large outbreak in the country:

> Ok, yes, I think first of all that the disease exists. Oh, yes, I think the disease exists. However, it did not start here, it started in China, and today it has attacked the whole world. I really do think the disease exists. But now, here [in Burkina Faso], seeing the things that are happening, it leaves us wanting more. Personally, it leaves me unsatisfied, because at the level of our rulers, there are things that are happening that put doubts in our heads.

When asked to explain this statement, he said:

> That is to say, given the reaction of our rulers, given everything that is currently happening in our country, it brings us to a certain level where

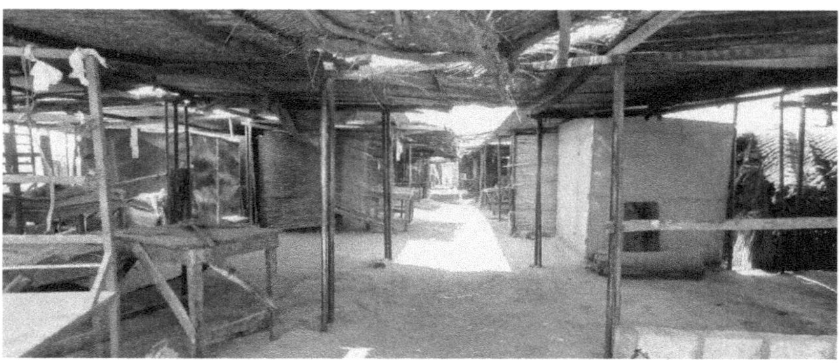

Figure 7.1. Empty market during lockdown, Burkina Faso (© Landry Bambara)

> we really wonder if the disease has really arrived in our country, or how it is. You see, we are asking many questions now about the disease.

When asked what the government had done that made him question whether COVID-19 existed in Burkina Faso, he elaborated by saying that people in the government contradict themselves.

Martin linked his doubts with his reservations about the government, hinting at contradictory statements by a couple of ministers concerning the recent death of a deputy member and whether it was related to COVID-19. Yaya, a 43 year old businessman, also expressed mistrust of the government's handling of the outbreak:

> Otherwise, the disease is there. I didn't say it wasn't, eh, it's there, but the government exaggerates the seriousness of this disease. The government has fooled us too much. The disease is not that alarming. It's not that alarming with us here. But they flattered us too much with that. It's not good. Explain the facts to us so that we understand. But to exaggerate the disease when it's not at all alarming, we really don't appreciate that. (Interview, 6 May 2020)

Yaya was very skeptical of the government, saying that by introducing many restrictions, the government only wanted to create panic in the population. Like other interlocutors, he highlighted that fact that he had not seen any individuals suffering from COVID-19: "I have watched on the television, their hospital Blaise Compaoré, they say that they are [hospitalized] there. I have seen that the president went there, but they have not shown any of the diseased." Soungalo, whom I quoted above, was very skeptical about the government's handling of the epidemic and was convinced that it was all about politics and money:

> Everyone can see that the government has dealt with this disease in a political way. He [the president] dealt with disease from the angle of politics and money. Since the disease arrived in Burkina, we hear about donations from here and there. We hear that one type of association has donated so and so many francs, another has donated 100 million, and that one bank has donated 200 million. All you hear about is money, donated money only. This is what leads me to think that the government sees this disease as a business. The president has even said that the diseased will be taken care of at the hotels and that this will cost 121 billion. People then criticized this, and they have reduced this to 57 billion. If you take decisions like that while the doctors were on strike for eight months due to lack of equip-

> ment at the hospitals, but the 121 billion could solve this problem and one would not have to use hotels for the diseased. (Interview, 6 May 2020)

Although one of the main priorities of the government's COVID-19 response plan was to develop an efficient communication strategy, many people expressed their doubts about the real intentions of the government. Although the government of Roch Marc Christian Kaboré was democratically elected in 2016 and reelected in 2020, popular support was not strong; the introduction of severe restrictions, which disrupted everyday life, particularly for urban citizens, seemed to weaken trust in the president and his government during these early months of the pandemic.

Restrictions

In a long message to the nation on 2 April 2020, a week after the implementation of restrictive measures, the president expressed his concern about the sacrifices citizens had to make in order to manage the pandemic, saying: "We are aware that the measures we take to slow down and combat the spread of COVID-19 have adverse effects on the daily lives of our fellow citizens, but they are essential if we want to break the chain of transmission of the virus." Then he continued the message listing a number of temporary tax alleviations and reductions in water and electricity bills. However, the closing down of the bigger markets and of borders, which hindered the import and export of goods from neighboring countries, had serious implications for millions of people in Burkina Faso. Souna, a forty-three-year-old hairdresser in Bobo-Dioulasso, said:

> In my opinion, we liked that the government took these measures. We liked the work they did. I would say that the government wanted to protect us from this disease. But it had consequences for us. It is true that the government protects us from this disease. But it is difficult for us. It is just so that we cannot shout for those people to hear. It's difficult. We beg them to help us. We are in difficulties. But, we cannot approach them to say how difficult it is for us. We are really in trouble. The measures he [the president] took are for us to have health. But what can we poor people say about it? We can't say anything. We just sit down to watch them. God will help us. Otherwise, we are in trouble. (Interview, 7 May 2020)

On the one hand, Souna appreciated that the government actually took action and introduced a number of protective measures.

On the other hand, she was discouraged about the fragile economic situation she and others were left with and their limited possibilities for communicating this to the government. Soulango, the wholesale dealer I quoted above, explained the disruption of his commercial activities:

> I can say that the closing down of the *grand marché* [the big market] for twenty-three days has really reduced the turnover of my business. Before, on a daily basis, I could have a turnover of about a million before their disease-story started. It varied, really. But my loss has been enormous due to the closing of the market. Furthermore, I have stock warehouses in addition to the warehouse at the market, where I have to pay a rent of more than 500,000. I was just sitting at home, and I really lost a lot.

It was also a very tough period for the many people who participate in the informal economy selling vegetables, fruits, and foodstuffs, as well as those involved in other small-scale commercial activities that depend on customers at the usually bustling marketplaces.

Kotim, who used to sell vegetables at the market, was very upset, saying: "If you don't sell anything, how will you eat? Will any of the rulers know me, and come and give me money? He [the president] does not know how it is at my house. The difficulties that I have, only I know how it is to live through those. He, he does not know that, because he already has what he likes. It is me who is in difficulties." She continued, saying: "It has caused me a lot of troubles, don't you see, I am sitting here going through my garlic. Everything is rotten, I meticulously go through it all and throw out" (Interview, 6 May 2020). Kotim was obviously not satisfied with the lockdown, as it hit her small business hard. In the quote above, she also alluded to the social distance between herself and the president and her feeling of being let down. Furthermore, many citizens living under precarious conditions did not have electricity or running water in their homes, and thus did not benefit from the compensation packages launched by the government.

Temporal Frictions

Despite a general trend of economic growth in Burkina Faso in the years before the pandemic, many households were highly vulnerable to food insecurity, and almost 60 percent of the population had difficulties meeting their basic caloric needs (World Bank 2018).

The lockdown hit hard and made it even more difficult for many families to provide for the next meal. By 20 April, after almost a month of lockdown, one big market in Ouagadougou (out of a total of forty markets) and one in Bobo-Dioulasso were reopened. Then, a group of merchants in Ouagadougou organized a protest against the restrictions, demanding the government reopen all markets in the city. Roadblocks using stones, used tires, and tree trunks were set up. The protestors said that they had nothing left to eat and that few people benefited from food donations. *Africanews* quoted one of the protestors, who claimed that the country would catch fire if the markets were not reopened and that the pandemic was being used politically.[16] Traders at other markets made similar assertions.[17] Many people were also upset about the ban on religious ceremonies in churches and mosques. The many protests forced the government to rethink the lockdown measures. In early May, the religious institutions were reopened, and the nightly curfew was lifted by 3 June 2020. However, primary and secondary schools remained closed until September 2020.

As described above, many people expressed ambiguity about the government's swift actions during the early phase of the pandemic. The invisibility of the disease—the fact that people had not seen actual cases of COVID-19—was an important issue. This, combined with the economic consequences of the lockdown and general disappointment with Kaboré's government, generated uncertainty and doubt about the severity of the situation. For many, COVID-19 was a "not-yet-present" disease. Its invisibility during these first months of the epidemic fueled a general skepticism about the need to introduce radical and restrictive measures. Based on experiences from other countries and on a multitude of mathematical models and scenarios, the government anticipated COVID-19's rapid spread and took immediate action in order to prevent a huge outbreak, which would have been extremely difficult for the unprepared and weak health system to handle.

The government struggled with the problem of time, having seen how quickly the pandemic moved across continents. Using the risk technologies proposed by WHO and other global institutions, the government made projections from the limited and fragmented data available. In her discussion about risk, uncertainty, and possibility, Louise Amoore defined a specific anticipatory logic: "it acts not strictly to *prevent* the playing out of a particular course of events on the basis of past data tracked forward into probable futures but to *preempt* an unfolding and emergent event in relation to an array of possible projected futures. It seeks not to forestall the future via calculation but to incorporate the very unknowability and profound uncertainty of the future into imminent decision" (2013: 9). Risk in the mode of possibility rather than strict probability, she says, "does not govern by the deductive proving or disproving of scientific and statistical data but by the inductive incorporation of suspicion, imagination, and preemption" (Amoore 2013: 10). The response plan developed by the government in March 2020 projected possible future scenarios in Burkina Faso, inductively forecasting worst case and most likely scenarios.

Anthony Giddens uses the notion of "time-space distanciation" in his characterization of modern social life. He defines this as a "condition under which time and space are organized so as to connect presence and absence" (Giddens 1990: 14). During the first phase of COVID-19 in Burkina Faso, we saw, as described above, a temporal disconnection between the government's anticipatory regime (Adams, Murphy, and Clarke 2009; Anderson 2010) and the local residents' demand for understanding in the actual present. This is what we have termed *temporal friction* (Samuelsen and Toé 2021). During the first few months, the government and the local residents of Bobo-Dioulasso did not relate to the "future" in the same way. Through the government's pre-emption, the future was brought into the present, but this was not a presence our interlocutors could recognize. They were positioned in "different time zones."

An Exceptional Epidemic

In our conversations with citizens in Bobo-Dioulasso in the first phase of the pandemic, many talked about COVID-19 as exceptional. Beatrice, who as a young child suffered from meningitis, was convinced that COVID-19 was a much more serious disease:

> I say it is a serious illness because immediately, if there is a case in this neighborhood, they are going to quarantine the whole neighborhood. We have to make a blockade for everyone who is here. Because you are not supposed to go out. They will say to stay at home. It's really a disease, which is not good, the stigma, because when I listen to the radio, when it

> is said that you have this, people will be afraid to approach you. And it is really not appreciated when you are isolated from your family. It's not like meningitis, where you are able to get visitors. This disease [COVID-19] is truly exceptional.

Later in the conversation, Beatrice returns to the exceptionality of COVID-19, highlighting that it affects the whole world, not only Burkina Faso (Interview, 13 June 2020).

Fatmata, a seventy-three-year-old housewife living in Bobo-Dioulasso, said: "This disease! There are all kinds of diseases that occur in the world, but since we were born, we have never seen this kind." After a short break, she continued:

> A disease evolves and we close the mosques, the markets, we don't sit next to each other, you don't talk to the person next to you, all the transport routes have been closed, no one can travel. We've never seen that before. We stopped going to the mosque for two months. You pray in your house at home. But I have never seen anybody here among us who were infected by this disease. They talk about it, but I have never heard of anybody who were infected. Here, in Bobo, it has infected somebody, or it has not infected anyone, I don't know. (Interview, August 2020)

Later in the conversation, Fatmata compares COVID-19 with previous epidemics, saying:

> This disease [COVID-19], here, they say that it is more serious. In Burkina, I have not heard that it is serious. But for the countries of the whites, we hear that it kills thousands of people. It seems that this disease is more serious. We have never heard of a serious disease like this disease; it's more serious than all these diseases [we know], because the two major diseases [AIDS and Ebola] I'm talking about, they haven't stopped people from doing anything. But this disease has prevented people from doing many things.

Fatmata refers to the fact that previous epidemics had not led to government restrictions like those during COVID-lockdown. When I asked Kotim how she perceived COVID-19, compared to previous epidemics, she replied:

> This one [COVID-19] is frightening us. AIDS killed people. We saw those people who contracted AIDS. At that time the mosques were not closed, the markets were not closed. Is this a good thing? Ebola came, did that close the mosques? The mosques were not closed, the markets were not closed. This . . . coronavirus, what is [it]? The markets are closed, the

> mosques are closed. And we have not even seen it with our own eyes. We have heard about it, but not seen it. Oh, this time, the president has given us a difficult task. This is not okay.[18]

Mariam, a young civil servant, highlights the particularity of COVID-19, saying:

> I take an example, like the coronavirus like that, it is said that we should avoid closeness, direct contact. This is why the government has taken action. Whereas at the time of meningitis, there was no such demands. It was a contagious disease, but there were no such measures as avoiding contact.

Since the disease itself remained invisible to most citizens, the exceptionality of COVID-19 was to a large extent related to the ways the government responded and in particular to the severe restrictions on people's social and economic life.

Experiencing COVID-19

In our COVID-19 field study in 2020 and 2021, we came across five people who had experienced COVID-19 themselves: four men and one woman from thirty-five to fifty-nine years old. Among the five, there was one health worker, one agricultural consultant, one businessman, one security guard at a mining company, and one housewife. Their stories of illness vary, from one who was asymptomatic to one who was hospitalized for twenty days. However, a common theme in all five narratives is that being diagnosed and then confined as part of the containment strategy was talked about very discreetly.

Yacouba, who worked as a security guard with a mining company located in the southwest, tested positive at a routine check. The employees were confined for a total of seven days before entering the mining area, with a test on the first and the sixth day. During the week of quarantine they stayed at a nearby hotel. After a positive test, Yacouba was isolated in a hotel room for twenty-four days, as the company wanted to see a confirmed negative test before ending the isolation. He remained asymptomatic for the whole period. He has, however, never told anyone about the positive test or the twenty-four days of isolation. He did not want to create panic in the family, he said. His older sister had just lost a child and had come to stay with him and his family to recover from the loss. He did not want to tell them about his diagnosis, being afraid that such a message would generate too much anxiety in the family. He was happy, though, that he had received his certificate (of the negative COVID-19 test) and said that eventually he would tell his wife and show her the certificate.

Amina was suffering from diabetes, and right from the start of the pandemic, she was told by family members that she should be extra careful, as they had heard that COVID-19 was more dangerous for people with diabetes. She became very afraid, she said, when the district hospital referred her to the Belle Ville (the COVID-19 center). At that time, she was very weak and needed extra oxygen; all the members of the family were crying, as they feared the COVID-19 diagnosis. The doctors never told her directly that she suffered from COVID-19, but she was given a single room at Belle Ville and her children were not allowed to visit her. She explained the doctors' "under-communication" in the following way:

> The doctors don't want to discourage a person, because even if the person is dying, they still give a prescription to go and buy medicine. Because they don't want to discourage anyone. So, if they tell me to go to this place and they say that it is these sick people who are there. That's when I got scared and started crying. I was very discouraged. I did not eat. All my children were discouraged.

The COVID-19 diagnosis was never communicated directly to her; the health staff only talked about her diabetes. However, since she was coughing and was referred to the COVID-19 center, both she and her children were convinced that she also suffered from COVID-19. In the other three cases, the COVID-19 diagnosis was also dealt with discreetly. Thus, this new epidemic not only remained invisible to most people, but was also muted, both by the patients themselves and by health staff.

Moments of State Presence

As demonstrated above, many people expressed frustration with the lockdown and severe restrictions during the first part of the epidemic. Many of these frustrations were directed toward the government, which was seen as distant and unaware of the reality of everyday life for ordinary citizens. Many had huge economic losses, and even though a number of initiatives were implemented to compensate for the loss of income, those initiatives did not really benefit people living in a day-to-day economy. However, over time, as case rates in Burkina remained relatively low and people did not see or know anyone suffering from COVID-19, we sensed a change of attitude toward the government's way of handling the epidemic, especially as people heard from the media about the pandemic's overwhelming impact on many countries in the Global North. In the interviews we conducted during August, September, and October 2020, people talked much more positively about the government's actions. David, a thirty-two-year-old sports coach, was impressed by the intensive information campaigns and compared them with the government's communication about previous epidemics, such as meningitis and measles, saying:

> There is a big difference. For example, meningitis, measles, there are epidemics in Burkina. But communication does not pass like the COVID. Communication is almost zero compared to the COVID. We are not going to see the government put out ads, send messages five, six times a day for another epidemic. But for the corona, it was rebroadcasted. There have been broadcasts; there have been reports. There was everything about it. It was live. They really maxed out.

Mohammad, a university student, said that in the beginning of the COVID-19 pandemic in Burkina Faso, he did not believe that it existed, and he did not follow the restrictions. Only when one of his friends from university who studied medicine told him that he should take it seriously did he begin to follow the public advice. In mid-August 2020, he said:

> We praise the government, because they have made an effort. It is a landlocked country, there is no money, and if we compare to Ivory Coast, it is not the same thing. Despite all of this, our government has swarmed to fight the disease. While the number of cases is still high in Côte d'Ivoire, we can say that the measures they [the Burkinabe government] took and the curfew they introduced paid off. It was not in vain. (Interview, 13 August 2020)

Michel, a twenty-year-old student, felt that the intense coverage of the COVID-19 outbreak in Burkina had been counterproductive because the daily announcement of the number of new cases had

PRIMATURE

SERVICE D'INFORMATION DU GOUVERNEMENT

BURKINA FASO
Unité-Progrès-Justice

Ouagadougou, le 15 avril 2020

Communiqué

Coronavirus (Covid-19) au Burkina Faso

A la date du **14 avril 2020**, la situation de la maladie à Coronavirus au Burkina Faso se présente comme suit :

- **123** échantillons analysés dont **64** cas suspects et **59** contrôles ;
- **14** nouveaux cas confirmés dont **11** à Ouagadougou et **03** à Bobo-Dioulasso ;
- **49** guérisons, portant à **226**, le total des guérisons ;
- **02** décès, portant à **32**, le total des décès ;
- **284** cas sous traitement.

Au total, 542 cas ont été confirmés dont 211 femmes et 331 hommes, depuis le 09 mars 2020.

Le gouvernement rappelle que la maladie à Coronavirus (Covid-19) est très contagieuse et que le respect des mesures barrières est essentiel pour interrompre la chaine de transmission.

La Coordonnatrice
Mafarma SANOGO
Chevalier de l'ordre national

Figure 7.2. Daily COVID-10 announcement, Ministry of Health, Burkina Faso

created too much fear. However, overall, he thought the government had managed the outbreak effectively, saying:

> They have done well. We saw that all the mosques were closed, all churches, all the bars. There were no gatherings. Everybody stayed at home by themselves. That was to protect us. It is true that it [the epidemic] is still here, but it is not like before. The government has done well.

Simon, a thirty-four-year-old teacher, compared the situation in Burkina Faso with that of neighboring countries, praising the government of Burkina Faso for its hard work to control the pandemic. He also emphasized that the government had put much more effort in controlling this epidemic compared to previous epidemics in order to act against the "global psychosis."

Many of the people we interviewed praised the government for its swift action and for introducing a number of seemingly effective restrictions to control the pandemic in Burkina Faso. By mid-August 2020, high levels of COVID-19 transmission appeared less likely. Some people compared Burkina Faso to neighboring countries with higher levels of COVID-19 transmission, and many were well aware of how dramatic the situation in the Global North had been, particularly in the early phase of the pandemic. Omar, who worked as a teacher in Bobo-Dioulasso, explained what happened when people began to realize that COVID-19 was not as dangerous a disease in Burkina Faso as first imagined: "According to me, the disease is still present. But now, we are not so interested in the disease anymore. Now, the fear is reduced, we now see that it is almost a disease like all the other diseases. So, it is not as deadly as it was first believed to be" (Interview, 21 September 2020). He complimented the government, saying that it did what it could to control the epidemic, but he also observed that sometimes the government's communication was not honest, that the figures presented were sometimes inconsistent. At the end of the interview, he expressed his hope that the government would mobilize the people around the problems of security and terrorism as they had mobilized around the pandemic: "My suggestion is that they have to think of mobilizing the population around terrorism, which is more serious than COVID-19. They only have to stimulate the solidarity of the Burkinabe so that each Burkinabe can contribute in the end, so that we end terrorism and find peace, freedom."

Conclusion

During the early phase of the pandemic in Burkina Faso, it was not the disease itself that caused disruption, but rather the restrictive measures that transformed the rhythm of everyday life (Trentmann 2020). Similar findings have been reported from other African countries (Manderson and Levine 2021; Parker, MacGregor, and Akello 2020). The pandemic lockdown also interrupted the "inertia of the present," as Josep Maria Antentas calls it (2020). As I described above, the pre-emptive lockdown strategy created frictions of temporality between ordinary citizens and the government. Time commonly understood as consisting of a past, present, and future was disrupted. According to Ann Game, "whether these elements are understood to be in a linear or non-linear relation, a disruption to the future implies an unsettling of the whole structure of relations" (1997: 117). However, this is not to say that disruptions are unusual in Burkina Faso. On the contrary, people are used to power cuts, water cuts, and other infrastructural breakdowns, and they are used to being flexible and adjusting routines and habits to changing conditions. During the lockdown period, many people, both rural and urban, displayed what Trentmann would call the "elasticity of the everyday rhythm" (Trentmann 2020).

However, for many people, particularly people living on a day-to-day income, the lockdown stretched this elasticity too far. Many simply could not afford the lockdown. During this period, skepticism about the actual existence (and severity) of the epidemic and about the government's handling of the situation was predominant. A desperate atmosphere emerged among small-scale business people, bar workers, and artists. However, as demonstrated above, the government was also praised for its actions and its apparent interest in caring for health of the population, particularly in the period after most of the lockdown measures were lifted. Years of disappointment with the government's failure of Blaise Compaoré and his successor, Roch Marc Kaboré, regarding their responsibility to care for the country's citizens was at least momentarily replaced by a popular recognition of the government's ability to manage a lurking pandemic. While the disease itself remained invisible to most people, the restrictive measures introduced by the government served as technologies of visibility. That is, the state exerted its presence through these interventions, which people eventually appreciated. Citizens also sensed that they were seen by the state—at least momentarily (Street 2012). The street demonstrations and protests against the lockdown of the markets in the major cities of Burkina Faso, including Bobo-Dioulasso, also served as technologies of visibility in a very literal sense.

Notes

1. For up-to-date information about COVID-19, see Johns Hopkins University & Medicine, "Coronavirus Resource Center." Retrieved 29 September 2022 from https://coronavirus.jhu.edu.
2. As explained in the introduction, this chapter is based on a series of conversations with forty-six citizens in Bobo-Dioulasso during 2020 as well as

information from newspapers, public announcements from the Ministry of Health, government plans and reports, and social media posts. Due to the tense security situation and COVID-19 restrictions, it has not been possible for me to visit the village of Keru during the pandemic. The conversations in Bobo-Dioulasso were planned and organized jointly by senior researcher Lea Paré Toé, research assistant Estelle Solange Toé, and myself. Estelle conducted the interviews. I thank Lea and Estelle for their permission to use the material in this chapter.

3. According to Joel Breman (2021), the Egyptian Pharaoh Ramses V died of smallpox in 1157 BCE.
4. Cotton Mather used his knowledge about inoculation during a smallpox outbreak in Boston in 1721, and although the inoculation technique continued to be controversial in Europe, quite a few of the elites were inoculated. The first smallpox vaccine was developed in 1800, and the disease was officially declared eradicated in 1980.
5. The program included seven countries in West Africa. Burkina Faso (then known as Upper Volta) was one of them, with around 80 percent of its territory included in the original Onchocerciasis Control Program.
6. In 2011, twenty cases of cholera were registered in Burkina Faso (Kaboré et al. 2018).
7. According to the World Bank, 88 percent of children aged 12 to 23 months are immunized against measles. World Bank, "Immunization, measles (% of children ages 12–23 months)—Burkina Faso." Retrieved 19 July 2023 from https://data.worldbank.org/indicator/SH.IMM.MEAS?locations=BF.
8. While prevalence rates in some countries in Southern Africa reached more than 30 percent for a number of years, it remained between 2 percent and 4 percent in Burkina Faso.
9. World Bank, "Prevalence of HIV, total (% of population ages 15–49)—Burkina Faso." Retrieved 19 July 2023 from https://data.worldbank.org/indicator/SH.DYN.AIDS.ZS?locations=BF.
10. The WHO declared COVID-19 "a public health emergency of international concern" (PHEIC) on 30 January 2020.
11. Afrique Données Recherche, "Cas et décès COVID-19 au Burkina Faso." Retrieved 19 July 2023 from https://www.COVID19afrique.com/burkina-faso.
12. The number of confirmed COVID-19 cases and COVID-19-related deaths varies depending on the source. In an official government announcement dated 12 April 2020, a total of 505 confirmed cases and 28 deaths (registered since 9 March 2020) were reported, which is fewer deaths than recorded in the World Bank report.
13. Actually, this response plan was a revised version of an existing epidemic response plan.
14. The list was expanded when new potential epidemic infections were added.
15. Many people, especially in the early phase of the pandemic, talked about COVID-19 as a new outbreak of a previous epidemic rather than as a completely new disease.

16. *Africanews*, "Burkinabe Traders Demonstrate to Demand Reopening of Markets," 28 April 2020. Retrieved 19 July 2023 from https://www.africanews.com/2020/04/28/burkinabe-traders-demonstrate-to-demand-reopening-of-markets.
17. Alice Suglimani Thiombiano, "COVID-19 au Burkina Faso: Les commerçants de Nabi-Yaar manifestent pour la réouverture du marché," *Burkina24*, 28 April 2020. Retrieved 19 July 2023 from https://burkina24.com/2020/04/28/COVID-19-au-burkina-faso-les-commercants-de-nabi-yaar-manifestent-pour-la-reouverture-du-marche.
18. See also Helle Samuelsen and Lea Paré Toé (2021) for a discussion of popular responses during the early phase of the COVID-19 pandemic in Burkina Faso. Some of the quotes in this chapter are also used there.

Conclusion

Fragile Futures

Citizens in Keru live precarious lives full of uncertainties, and the state is in many ways marginal to their everyday lives. It is obvious to me, after following Thomas and his family for more than two decades, that rural families orient themselves toward the future, both the immediate future and the future of the coming generations, in many of their everyday decisions and activities. They invest a lot of energy and work in preventive and therapeutic activities in cases of sickness, and they search for a range of opportunities to supplement their income, from growing vegetables for the local market to high-risk migration. However, the overall situation in the country, particularly for rural citizens, is becoming more perilous as the increasing population exerts pressure on land, seasonal rainfall becomes more and more unpredictable due to climate change, and public services, such as local police and health care, remain consistently absent. Over time, I have of course also noticed positive changes in Keru, such as the establishment of a new dispensary—now with electricity—and a new school serving the growing number of children in the village. The rapid diagnostic test for malaria was introduced as a new technology at the local dispensary, and free health care is available for children under five and pregnant women. Furthermore, many families, though far from all, have managed to improve the quality of their housing through remittances from relatives, and most people now have access to a mobile phone.

While Thomas and his family had experienced many setbacks, the death of Caroline's son only one among many tragedies, the family was moving forward. When I saw Thomas in 2019, he told me, with a smile on his face, that one daughter was married with six children, another daughter was working in the public health care system, his elder son was almost ready to take responsibility for the family's farming activities, his younger son would hopefully soon return from Libya, and his two youngest daughters were pursuing further education. While this was good news, everyday life in rural Burkina Faso continues to be characterized by poverty and recurrent illness, especially for young children. In addition, the young people of Keru look into an uncertain and fragile future where it will be impossible for most to live as subsistence farmers and difficult for most to get stable jobs, either within Burkina Faso or as migrant workers. The elderly, like Thomas and Beatrice, also worry about their future. Who is going to take care of them when they are no longer able to work? Who will be able to take over as head of household and ensure support for the family and the community? At the village level, despite a number of improvements, basic living conditions have not changed radically over the last twenty years.

With inspiration from Paul Ricoeur and others, I have used fragility, care, responsibility, and hope as central concepts in all three parts of this book. The notion of fragility relates to the future: something fragile might easily break or chip, thus it is also about contingency, uncertainty, and insecurity. The people of Keru work actively to sustain and improve their living conditions and to secure a safe and thriving future for the coming generations. I focused, first, on family care and everyday life. I explored how the therapeutic pathways of the mothers move back and forth between home treatment, advice sought from local healers, and visits to the public biomedical facilities. I also examined how embarking on a migrant *aventure* is to be seen a form of care work filled with hopes and aspirations, both for those leaving the village as well as for those staying behind. I then analyzed how care technologies were used to nurse relationships between humans as well as between humans and non-humans. In the last part of the book, I zoomed in on the government institutions that are supposed to provide care for the public with a particular focus on the rural dispensary and the routine practice of diagnosing malaria in most cases of fever. With scarce diagnostic equipment and modest capacity, frontline health workers have little to offer. In the last chapter, using data collected during the pandemic in Bobo-Dioulasso, I zoom out from the village of Keru to a focus on how the COVID-19 pandemic affected state-citizen dynamics.

I have examined ambiguities of care in different contexts, emphasizing the multiple dimensions of care, including the work of "caring for" someone as well as the affective implications of "caring about" someone and nurturing social relations. Care is omnipresent. Ontologically speaking, care is a core element of most social relationships, and, as Jessica Cooper suggests, it may be useful to think of it as a theory rather than as a concept.[1] I use the term *chronicity* to stress the long-term aspects of sickness and disease (Manderson et al. 2010). We are beyond the old dichotomy between acute infectious diseases, on the one hand, and non-communicable, chronic diseases on the other. In the introduction to *Chronic Conditions, Fluid States*, Lenore Manderson and Carolyn Smith-Morris emphasize that "the distinctions between chronic and acute, communicable and non-communicable are social facts" (Manderson and Smith-Morris 2010: 3). Those distinctions become blurred when common infectious diseases that are, in principle, curable become chronic. In this region, many infections persist, and the health of many small children fluctuates between minor improvements and relapses in a continuous loop during most of their childhood. The idea of "everyday emergencies" is not an oxymoron; rather, it designates the chronic acuteness of child health in this part of the world. As we have seen in the preceding chapters, conditions of uncertainty can be productive as they present opportunities for the future. The pragmatic "trying again" and the persistent tinkering described here are gestures of care that actively attend to these openings in the search for a good life (Mol 2008).

The Absent-Present State

As mentioned in the introduction, Burkina Faso has over the last eight to ten years become an extremely unstable place. Numerous terrorist attacks, both in the border areas and in the central part of the country, have undermined citizens' trust in the government's capacity to provide basic protection and a minimum level of public services, making the country increasingly fragile. The popular insurrection in 2014 leading to the end of Blaise Compaoré's twenty-seven-year-long presidency propelled a more outspoken popular critique of governance and public services. Furthermore, a stream of self-defense groups called *Koglweogo* (from Mooré: *Kogle*, "to protect," + *weogo*, "bush land") have emerged in most parts of the country, both urban and rural, over a relatively short period. The members of these militia-like units are local volunteers, primarily young men (Hagberg 2019). With a weakened state, a critical security situation, and increasing inequality, the outlook for improving the health of the population is bleak, and the younger generations are left with few chances of obtaining a future in which they are able to get an education, find a job, and sustain a decent livelihood.

As discussed, the security situation has for years been a huge problem for the government. There have been numerous attacks on government buildings, including military barracks, schools, and dispensaries; these attacks have led to many military and civilian casualties, particularly in the northern and eastern provinces, and contributed to a further destabilization of the country. As mentioned earlier, a coup d'état took place in January 2022, with Colonel Damiba as the front figure. The momentary popularity of Roch Marc Kaboré's government that emerged after the first phase of COVID-19 was not sustained, and on the day of the military coup many people went into the streets to celebrate, expressing hope for a new regime that could stop the terrorism and regain control of the whole country. A second military coup took place just nine months after Colonel Damiba's coup, this time led by Captain Ibrahim Traoré, who hailed from another section of the military. The two military coups in 2022 exemplify the extremely tenuous security situation. Part of the country is controlled by various jihadist groups, and the fact that both military coups were largely welcomed by the population during the first months of both coups is probably due to both a real and concrete fear of ongoing jihadist terrorism and a fatigue after years of feeling betrayed by poor governments.

For many of Keru's residents, the state is both present and absent. It is present in the sense that everybody knows who the president is. Blaise Compaoré was recognized as a very powerful man during his many years as president, and citizens were fully engaged in discussions about the future of the country during the 2015 and 2020 presidential elections following Compaoré's ouster (Hagberg, Kibora, Ouattara et al. 2015; Hagberg, Kibora, Barry et al. 2019). During the COVID-19 pandemic, residents in Bobo-Dioulasso praised the government for showing statecraft (at least at the time when the most severe restrictions were lifted). The state is also present in the sense that public institutions are physically located in the village and staffed with government representatives. At the same time, the state exists primarily as an absence. Alice Street explains this phenomenon in her study of Madang Hospital in Papua New Guinea: "The state is not imagined as an abstract entity but as an urban elite of politicians and administrators who have little interest in bringing governance, and associated 'development' to the nation's rural inhabitants" (Street 2012: 12). Furthermore, most government institutions in the rural areas of Burkina Faso are characterized by emptiness and absenteeism. The absence of diagnostic equipment means frontline health care workers have to make decisions on the basis of clinical experience and "guesswork and contingency," as Gupta would likely put it (Gupta 2012: 14).

Viewing the dispensary, a biomedical government institution, as one of the few "spaces of encounter" (Obadare and Adebanwi 2010: 2) between rural citizens and the state allows us to tell a story of everyday health care practices that includes much more than the clinic, which is just one of many stakeholders in the field of health care. Families, particularly mothers of sick children, seek care and treatment in this medical field by juggling various options rather than by making strategic decisions. Families actively explore a "field of action" in which they seek ways to improve their health and diversify their livelihood. Looking at the state (and its representatives) from a perspective outside state institutions contributes, I hope, to theorizing about the citizen-state relationship. Rural citizens are marginal to the state (in the sense that the quality of state services thins out with distance from the central institutions), but, as discussed here, the state also becomes marginal to the rural population through its continued incapacity to deliver basic health care services, security, and prospects for an improved livelihood. Still, the state is an object of desire, in both rural and urban Burkina Faso: fewer infrastructural disruptions, better health services, and care for the public. And many parents hope, like Thomas and Beatrice, that at least one of their children will pass the test and become a government civil servant.

Perspectives for Global Health

From the margins of the state, outside of the biomedical institutions, the absence of the state becomes visible. Although the nearest biomedical health facility is located in the village itself, many preventive and therapeutic health care practices take place outside of those facilities. I do not have quantitative data about how often people visit non-biomedical practitioners or how many cases of sickness are treated solely at home, but my many conversations with mothers of sick children indicate that only a fraction of cases are brought to biomedical facilities for consultation. My examination of the therapeutic itineraries in Keru demonstrates the importance of understanding the diversity of human practice and experience within the domain of health through a renewed focus on treatment seeking in medical anthropology that includes both vernacular healing by local experts and self-treatment at home, as China Scherz suggests (2018). This suggestion follows the slow research movement introduced by Vincanne Adams and her colleagues, who underline that slow research takes the local as its starting point. "This 'local' can only be accessed through extended interaction in particular sites, what Joao Biehl calls 'on the ground'" (Adams, Burke, and Whitmarsh 2014: 182; Biehl 2007:109). I have done that through my focus on one rural village and one particular family within this village. I hope that studies like this will contribute constructively to the wider debates and discussions within medical anthropology and global health about the relationship between the local and the global. At the same time, I sympathize with Nolwazi Mkhwanazi's plea to medical anthropologists to be mindful about how we use the singular story, as it risks creating stereotypes (Mkhwanazi 2016). Drawing on the writer Chimamanda Ngozi Adichie, Mkhwananzi says that the problem with stereotypes is not that they are untrue but that they are incomplete. I am aware that my story about the village of Keru and Thomas's family is incomplete, yet I think that the "slow research" approach, where the single stories of the local are always examined in a wider context in which the entanglements between the local and the global are central, has the potential to enrich research in medical anthropology and global health. As Vicanne Adams Nancy Burke, and Ian Whitmarsh explain, the "local" is a term "that identifies the interaction of international, national, regional, neighborhood, and familial institutions as they coalesce and become visible" (2014: 182). Focusing on everyday health care practices in a community like Keru through the lens of one particular family and their neighbors over decades is based on a recognition that "local contexts matter" (Adams, Burke, and Whitmarsh 2014:

183), especially when situated within the wider social, political, and security context of Burkina Faso and the Central Sahel.

Viewing Burkina Faso's primary health care facilities as a critical "outsider," as presented here, is important, but admittedly also easy. This book does not focus on the everyday decisions health workers make during consultations with patients, their frustrations about an unstable flow of medicine, or the stress caused by mountains of paperwork and overly optimistic treatment targets (Pare Toe and Samuelsen 2020). Nor do I examine the "backstage" stories of donor dependency, political entanglements, corruption (REN-LAC 2018), or lack of resources in the educational system for effectively training health care workers. The challenges of providing decent primary health care to the Burkinabe population are enormous. It is my hope, though, that this book will contribute to bringing an "on the ground" perspective to the fore.

Furthermore, the fact that Burkina Faso follows the global trend of collecting and using (often unreliable) data should caution us. The increased datafication of health (Ruckenstein and Schüll 2017; Hutchinson et al. 2018) and the push for national and global metrics should be critically examined so long as the quality of health system data on consultations, diagnostics, and treatment is poor, as is often the case in Burkina Faso and other parts of Africa. I have critically discussed the high proportion of malaria diagnoses at the rural health facilities in Keru and neighboring villages, as it leaves many other health problems invisible. At the same time, I am, of course, fully aware that prioritization is necessary in under-resourced health systems.

During the writing of this book, the COVID-19 pandemic emerged. As discussed above, the pandemic event with the lockdown of many economic and social activities not only disrupted everyday life but also interrupted the "inertia of the present," to use Josep Maria Antentas's (2020) phrase. As I described above, it created temporal frictions between ordinary citizens and the government. The framing of an epidemic as exceptional or different from other epidemics (and thereby justifying exceptional responses) may have both positive and negative impacts on people's health and financial well-being. For example, emphasizing the fight against Ebola in West Africa at the expense of other health programs resulted in an increase in malaria and other infectious diseases, as well as disruptions in tuberculosis and antiretroviral treatments and low use of health facilities during the epidemic (Elston et al. 2017; Gomez Temesio 2018; Larkan, Ryan, and Kevany 2015). Furthermore, the deployment of the military in Sierra Leone during the Ebola epidemic to enforce restrictions as part of the control strategy weakened the relationship between citizens and the government (Benton 2017; Enria 2019). In Burkina Faso, the government did not use the military to put the COVID-19 restrictions into effect, and although many people appreciated the government's swift reaction to the pandemic, the relationship between citizens and the state continued to be challenged by the deteriorating security situation in the country.

Furthermore, while following the management of the epidemic at distance (Samuelsen and Toé 2021), it became clear to me that the health care system in Burkina Faso, as in many other countries, was not well prepared to prevent and control emerging epidemics. Burkina Faso has experienced severe health crises in the past, including recurrent measles and meningococcal epidemics, and the Ebola outbreak in neighboring countries challenged the whole region. These, together with the COVID-19 pandemic, have spurred the government to strengthen its infectious disease surveillance system (C.O. Diallo et al. 2022). It will require long-lasting and unprecedented political and economic commitments to reach the country's own ambitions of working to "build in 25 years, another and better Burkina Faso where the population will have achieved physical, mental and material development and improved general quality of life for all."[2] Even the most optimistic assessment would not expect this goal, first stated in 2005, to be fulfilled by 2030. The then minister of health, Professor Charlemagne Ouédraogo, announced in the spring of 2021 that a new plan for public health care in Burkina Faso was to be developed, to be known as the "Plan national de développement sanitaire (PNDS) 2021–2030." When announcing this new initiative, he declared that the period from 2021 to 2030 constitutes a challenge for his ministry, "in terms of resilience and strengthening of the health system and in strengthening the social dialogue and cohesion in order to be able to succeed in its mission, which is to guarantee a better state of health to the population."[3]

Despite massive structural challenges, families and individual family members continue to look for openings and opportunities as they engage with the many uncertainties they encounter in their

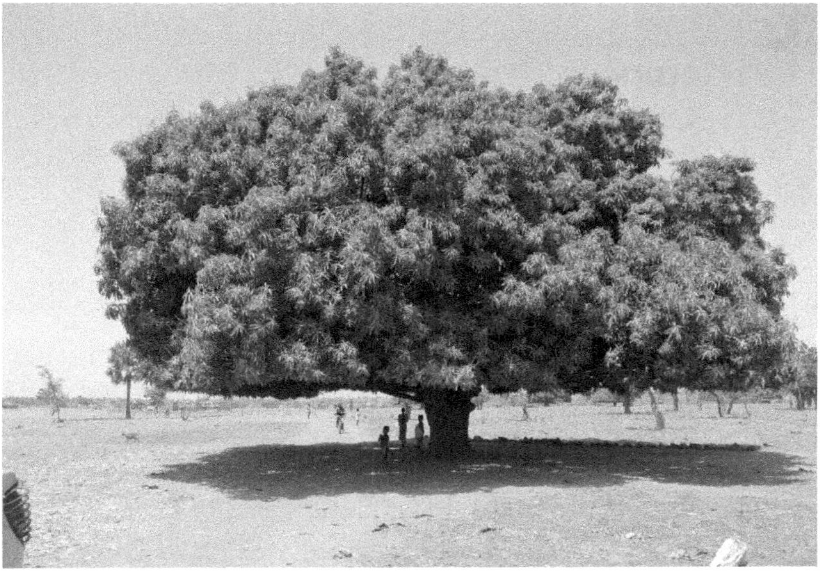

Figure 8.1. *Abre de palabre* (discussion tree), rural Burkina Faso (© Helle Samuelsen 2023)

everyday life. My purpose in offering a glimpse into the lives of Thomas and Beatrice and their seven children has been to provide an ethnographic account of how rural citizens navigate the health care system and how they strive with "open-ended hope" toward a good life in a context of multilevel fragility.

Notes

1. This was discussed by Jessica Cooper at a research seminar at the University of Copenhagen, 18 May 2021, where a parallel was drawn to Michel Foucault's theory of power.
2. "Etude Nationale Prospective 'Burkina 2025'" Rapport Generale, Conseil National de Prospective et de la Planification Stratégique (April 2005).
3. Ministère de la Santé, "Plan national de développement sanitaire," 10 February 2021. Retrieved 19 July 2023 from https://www.sante.gov.bf/detail?tx_news_pi1%5Baction%5D=detail&tx_news_pi1%5Bcontroller%5D=News&tx_news_pi1%5Bnews%5D=449&cHash=6e74b9a41b63a4b2ca1cd332a947bf77.

References

Adams, Vincanne, ed. 2016. *Metrics: What Counts in Global Health, Critical Global Health*. Durham, NC: Duke University Press.

Adams, Vincanne, Nancy J. Burke, and Ian Whitmarsh. 2014. "Slow Research: Thoughts for a Movement in Global Health." *Medical Anthropology* 33(3): 179–97.

Adams, Vincanne, Michelle Murphy, and Adele E Clarke. 2009. "Anticipation: Technoscience, Life, Affect, Temporality." *Subjectivity* 28: 246–65.

Adebanwi, Wale. 2022. *Everyday State and Democracy in Africa*. Columbus: Ohio State University.

Agamben, Giorgio. 1998. *Homo Sacer : Sovereign Power and Bare Life*. Stanford, CA: Stanford University Press.

Ajefu, Joseph B., and Joseph O. Ogebe. 2021. "The Effects of International Remittances on Expenditure Patterns of the Left-Behind Households in Sub-Saharan Africa." *Review of Development Economics* 25(1): 405–29.

Alber, Erdmute, and Heike Drotbohm. 2015. *Anthropological Perspectives on Care: Work, Kinship, and the Life-Course*. Houndmills: Palgrave Macmillan.

Alvar-Beltrán, Jorge, Abdalla Dao, Anna Dalla Marta, Ana Heureux, Jacob Sanou, and Simone Orlandini. 2020. "Farmers' Perceptions of Climate Change and Agricultural Adaptation in Burkina Faso." *Atmosphere* 11(8): 827.

Amoore, Louise. 2013. *The Politics of Possibility: Risk and Security beyond Probability*. Durham, NC: Duke University Press.

Anderson, Ben. 2010. "Preemption, Precaution, Preparedness: Anticipatory Action and Future Geographies." *Progress in Human Geography* 34(6): 777–98.

Antentas, Josep Maria. 2020. "Notes on Corona Crisis and Temporality." *Dialectical Anthropology* 44(3): 315–18.

Arendt, Hannah. 2013. *The Human Condition*. Chicago: University of Chicago Press.

Atkinson, Paul. 2007. *Ethnography: Principles in Practice*. London: Routledge.

Auyero, Javier. 2012. *Patients of the State: The Politics of Waiting in Argentina*. Durham, NC: Duke University Press.

Awumbila, Mariama. 2018. "Dynamics of Intra-Regional Migration in West Africa: Implications for ECOWAS Migration Policy." In *Migration in a Globalizing World: Perspectives from Ghana*, ed. Mariama Awumbila, Delali Badasu, and Joseph Teye, 9–30. Legon-Accra, Ghana: Sub-Saharan Publishers.

Azevedo, Mario J. 2017. "Africa's Health System (S) Performance on the Millennium Development Goals (Mdgs)." In *Historical Perspectives on the State of Health and Health Systems in Africa*, vol. II, African Histories and Modernities, 75–111. Cham: Palgrave Macmillan.

Babcock-Abrahams, Barbara. 1975. "'A Tolerated Margin of Mess': The Trickster and His Tales Reconsidered." *Journal of the Folklore Institute* 11(3): 147–86.

Badini, Amadé. 1994. *Naître et grandir chez les Moosé traditionnels: Découvertes du Burkina* [Born and raised among the traditional Moosé: Discoveries from Burkina]. Paris: SÉPIA A.D.D.B.

Bambio, Yiriyibin, and Salima Bouayad Agha. 2018. "Land Tenure Security and Investment: Does Strength of Land Right Really Matter in Rural Burkina Faso?" *World Development* 111: 130–47.

Banerjee, Abhijit, and Esther J. Duflo. 2006. "Addressing Absence." *Journal of Economic Perspectives* 20(1): 117–12.

Barnes, Marian. 2012. *Care in Everyday Life: An Ethic of Care in Practice*. Bristol: Brisol University Press. https://doi.org/10.1332/policypress/9781847428233.001.0001.

Belesova, Kristine, Christoph Gornott, James Milner, Ali Sié, Rainer Sauerborn, and Paul Wilkinson. 2019. "Mortality Impact of Low Annual Crop Yields in a Subsistence Farming Population of Burkina Faso under the Current and a 1.5° C Warmer Climate in 2100." *Science of the Total Environment* 691: 538–48.

Beneria, Lourdes, and Gita Sen. 1981. "Accumulation, Reproduction, and Women's Role in Economic Development: Boserup revisited." *Signs: Journal of Women in Culture and Society* 7(2): 279–98.

Benton, Adia. 2017. "Whose Security?: Militarization and Securitization During West Africa's Ebola Outbreak." In *The Politics of Fear: Médecins sans Frontières and the West African Ebola Epidemic*, ed. Michiel Hofman and Sokhieng Au, 25–50. Oxford: Oxford University Press.

Benton, Adia, Thurka Sangaramoorthy, and Ippolytos Kalofonos. 2017. "Temporality and Positive Living in the Age of HIV/AIDS: A Multi-Sited Ethnography." *Current Anthropology* 58(4): 454.

Benzein, Eva, Astrid Norberg, and Britt-Inger Saveman. 2001. "The Meaning of the Lived Experience of Hope in Patients with Cancer in Palliative Home Care." *Palliative Medicine* 15(2): 117–26.

Besarabic, Ana Lazara. 2020. "Disclosable Version of the ISR-Burkina Faso COVID-19 Preparedness and Response Project-P173858-Sequence No: 01." Washington, DC: World Bank Group. Retrieved 19 July 2023 from http://documents.worldbank.org/curated/en/270201600252911761/Disclosable-Version-of-the-ISR-Burkina-Faso-COVID-19-Preparedness-and-Response-Project-P173858-Sequence-No-01.

Biehl, João. 2005. "Technologies of Invisibility: Politics of Life and Social Inequality." *and Life Politics*, ed. Jonathan Xavier Inda. 248–271. Malden, MA: Blackwell Publishing.

———. 2007. *Will to Live: AIDS, Theapires and the Politics of Survival*. Princeton, NJ: Princeton University Press.

Biehl, João, and Adriana Petryna. 2013. *When People Come First: Critical Studies in Global Health*. Princeton, NJ: Princeton University Press.

Bierschenk, Thomas, and Jean-Pierre Olivier de Sardan. 2014. *States at Work*. Leiden, Netherlands: Brill.

Birungi, Harriet. 1998. "Injections and Self-Help: Risk and Trust in Ugandan Health Care." *Social Science & Medicine* 47(10): 1455–62.

Birungi, Harriet. and Susan Reynolds Whyte. 1994. "Injections in Uganda—Cause for Concern." *Essential Drugs Monitor* (18): 11.

Bisoffi, Zeno, Bienvenu Sodiomon Sirima, Andrea Angheben, Claudia Lodesani, Federico Gobbi, Halidou Tinto, and Jef Van den Ende. 2009. "Rapid Malaria Diagnostic Tests Vs. Clinical Management of Malaria in Rural Burkina Faso: Safety and Effect on Clinical Decisions. A Randomized Trial." *Tropical Medicine & International Health* 14(5): 491–98. https://doi.org/10.1111/j.1365-3156.2009.02246.x.

Bjarnesen, Jesper. 2013. "Diaspora at Home?: Wartime Mobilities in the Burkina Faso-Côte D'Ivoire Transnational Space." Ph.D. dissertation. Uppsala: Acta Universitatis Upsaliensis.

Bjertrup, Pia Juul. 2021. "(In) Visible Disease: Motions and Emotions Engendered by Papers and Diagnostics of People Accessing Healthcare in Burkina Faso." *Medicine Anthropology Theory* 8(3): 1–20.

Blom Hansen, Thomas, and Stepputat, Finn, eds. 2001. *States of Imagination. Ethnographic Explorations of the Postcolonial State*. Durham, NC: Duke University Press.

Bonko, Massa dit Achille, Francois Kiemde, Marc Christian Tahita, Palpouguini Lompo, Athanase M. Some, Halidou Tinto, Michael Boele van Hensbroek, Petra F. Mens, Henk D. F. H. Schallig. 2019. "The Effect of Malaria Rapid Diagnostic Tests Results on Antimicrobial Prescription Practices of Health Care Workers in Burkina Faso." *Annals of Clinical Microbiology and Antimicrobials* 18(1): 5.

Bonnet, Doris, 1988. *Corps biologique. Corps social. Procréation et maladies de l'enfant en pays mossi, Burkina Faso*. Paris : ORSTOM. Institut Français de recherche scientifique pour le développement en copération.

Borisenkova, Anna J 2012. "Introduction: Philosophical Anthropology and Social Analysis." *Études Ricoeuriennes/Ricoeur Studies* 3(1): 1–5.

Börzel, Tanja A., and Thomas Risse. 2021. *Effective Governance under Anarchy: Institutions, Legitimacy, and Social Trust in Areas of Limited Statehood*. Cambridge: Cambridge University Press.

Boserup, Esther. 1970. *Woman's Role in Economic Development*. London: George Allen & Unwin.

———. 1980. "The Position of Women in Economic Production and in the Household, with Special Reference to Africa." *The Household, Women and Agricultural Development. Miscellaneous Papers* 17: 11–16.

Bouchard, Michel 2011. "The State of the Study of the State in Anthropology." *Reviews in Anthropology* 40(3): 183–209.

Bourdieu, Pierre. 1990a. *In Other Words: Essays towards a Reflexive Sociology*. Stanford, CA: Stanford University Press.

———. 1990b. *The Logic of Practice*. Stanford, CA: Stanford University Press.

Breman, Joel G. 2021. "Smallpox Eradication: African Origin, African Solutions, and Relevance for Covid-19." *The American Journal of Tropical Medicine and Hygiene* 104(2): 416.

Brown, H., and A. H. Kelly. 2014. "Material Proximities and Hotspots: Toward an Anthropology of Viral Hemorrhagic Fevers." *Medical Anthropology Quarterly* 28(2): 280–303. https://doi.org/10.1111/maq.12092.

Brunsson, Nils, and Bengt Jacobsson. 2000. *A World of Standards*. Oxford: Oxford University Press.

Buckley, Anthony D. 1985. *Yoruba Medicine*. Oxford: Clarendon Press Oxford.

Caduff, Carlo. 2015. *The Pandemic Perhaps: Dramatic Events in a Public Culture of Danger*. Berkeley: University of California Press.

Carney, Eoin. 2015. "Depending on Practice: Paul Ricoeur and the Ethics of Care." *Les ateliers de l'éthique* 10(3): 29–48. https: //doi.org/10.7202/1037650ar.

Cartry, Michel. 1979. "Du village à la brousse ou le retour de la question: A propos des Gourmantché du Gobnangou (Haute-Volta)" [From the village to the bush or the return of the question: About the Gourmantché of Gobnangou (Upper Volta)]. In *La fonction symbolique: Essais d'anthropologie*, compiled by M. Izard and P. Smith, 265–88. Paris: Gallimard.

Chandler, Clare I. R., and Uli Beisel. 2017. "The Anthropology of Malaria: Locating the Social." *Medical Anthropology* 36(5): 411–21. https://doi.org/10.1080/01459740.2017.1306858.

Chandler, Clare, James Fairhead, Ann Kelly, Melissa Leach, Frederick Martineau, Esther Mokuwa, Melissa Parker, Paul Richards, and Annie Wilkinson. 2015. "Ebola: Limitations of Correcting Misinformation." *Lancet* 385(9975): 1275–77. https://doi.org/10.1016/S0140-6736(14)62382-5.

Charmillot, Maryvonne. 1997. *Les savoirs de la maladie: de l'éducation à la santé en contexte africain* [Knowledge of illness: From health education in the African context]. Geneva: Université de Genève Faculté de psychologie et des sciences de l'éducation.

Chigudu, Simukai 2019. "The Politics of Cholera, Crisis and Citizenship in Urban Zimbabwe: 'People Were Dying Like Flies.'" *Journal of African Affairs* 118(472): 413–34.

Cissao, Yacouba. 2019. "La Gestion des Conflits dans le Département de Tenkodogo (Burkina Faso): Entre Besoin et Rejet de l'Ètat." *NZASSA Revue Scientifique des Lettres, Langues et Arts, Littèratures et Civilisations, Sciences Humaines et Sociales, Communication* (2): 331–42.

———. 2020. "'Paka Constitution': Le Pragmatisme Des Représentants De l'État Burkinabè Dans La Gestion Des Conflits Locaux" ["Paka Constitution": The pragmatism of Burkinabè state representatives in the management of local conflicts.] *Mande Studies* 22(1): 121–43.

Colvin, Christopher J., Helen J. Smith, Alison Swartz, Jill W. Ahs, Jodie de Heer, Newton Opiyo, Julia C. Kim, Toni Marraccini, and Asha George. 2013. "Understanding Careseeking for Child Illness in Sub-Saharan Africa: A Systematic Review and Conceptual Framework Based on Qualitative Research of

Household Recognition and Response to Child Diarrhoea, Pneumonia and Malaria." *Social Science & Medicine* 86: 66–78.

Conrad Suso, Catherine T. 2020. "Involuntary Immobility and the Unfulfilled Rite of Passage: Implications for Migration Management in the Gambia, West Africa." *International Migration* 58(4): 184–94.

Cross, Hannah. 2020. "The Burkina Faso–Côte d'Ivoire Migration Corridor." In *Routledge Handbook of Migration and Development*, ed. Tanja Bastia and Ronald Skeldon, 469–473. Abigdon: Routledge.

Das, Veena, and Clara Han. 2015. *Living and Dying in the Contemporary World: A Compendium*. Berkeley: University of California Press.

Das, Veena, and Deborah Poole. 2004a. "State and Its Margins: Comparative Ethnographies." In *Anthropology in the Margins of the State*, ed. Veena Das and Deborah Poole, 3–33. Santa Fe: School of American Research Press.

Dauenhauer, Bernard P. 1986. *The Politics of Hope*. New York: Routledge & Kegan Paul.

de Certeau, Michel. 1988. *The Practice of Everyday Life*, trans. Steven Rendall. Berkeley: University of California Press.

Dettwyler, Katherine M. 1993. *Dancing Skeletons: Life and Death in West Africa*. Long Grove, IL: Waveland Press.

DHS, MEASURE. 2010. "Enquête Dèmographique et de Santé (EDS—IV) et à Indicateurs Multiples (MICS) EDSBF-MICS IV." Ministère de l'Economie et des Finances.

DHS+, Institut National de la Statistique et de la Démographie, and MEASURE. 2000. "Burkina Faso: Enqûete Démographique et de Santé 1998–99." Ministère de l'Économie et des Finances & Macro International Inc.

Diallo, Abdoulaye Hama, Nicolas Meda, Emmanuel Zabsonré, Halvor Sommerfelt, Simon Cousens, Thorkild Tylleskär, and PROMISE-EBF study group. 2010. "Perinatal Mortality in Rural Burkina Faso: A Prospective Community-Based Cohort Study." *BMC Pregnancy and Childbirth* 10(1): 45.

Diallo, Adama, Adjima Combary, Vanessa Veronese, Désiré Lucien Dahourou, Salifou Ouédraogo, Isidore Tiandiogo Traoré, and Corinne Simone Merle. 2022. "Delays in TB Diagnosis and Treatment Initiation in Burkina Faso during the COVID-19 Pandemic." *Tropical Medicine and Infectious Disease* 7(9): 237.

Diallo, Cheick Omar, Karin Linda Schiøler, Helle Samuelsen, and Koine Maxime Drabo. 2022. "Information System as Part of Epidemic Management in Burkina Faso: From Plan to Reality (Field Findings)." *BMC Public Health* 22(1): 1–13.

Dilger, Hansjörg, and Ute Luig, eds. 2010. *Morality, Hope and Grief: Anthropologies of AIDS in Africa*. New York: Berghahn.

Echenberg, Myron. 2011. *Africa in the Time of Cholera: A History of Pandemics from 1817 to the Present*, vol. 114. Cambridge: Cambridge University Press.

Ecks, Stefan. 2020. "Lockdowns Save, Lockdowns Kill: Valuing Life after Coronashock." *Somatosphere, Series: Dispatches from the Pandemic* 24 April. Retrieved 19 July 2023 from http://somatosphere.net/2020/lockdowns-save-lockdowns-kill-valuing-life-after-coronashock.html/.

Einarsdóttir, Jónína. (2000) 2004. *Tired of Weeping: Mother Love, Child Death and Poverty in Guinea-Bissau*. Madison: The University of Wisconsin Press.
Elston, James W. T., Christopher Cartwright, Patricia Ndumbi, and John Wright. 2017. "The Health Impact of the 2014–15 Ebola Outbreak." *Public Health* 143: 60–70.
Engberg-Pedersen, Lars, Louise Andersen, and Finn Stepputat. 2008. "Fragile Situations: Current Debates and Central Dilemmas." In *DIIS Report*. Copenhagen: Danish Institute for International Studies.
Enria, Luisa. 2019. "The Ebola Crisis in Sierra Leone: Mediating Containment and Engagement in Humanitarian Emergencies." *Development and Change* 50(6): 1602–23.
Erikson, Susan. 2016. "Metrics and Market Logics of Global Health." In *Metrics: What Counts in Global Health*, ed. Vincanne Adams, 147–62. Durham, NC: Duke University Press.
———. 2018. "Cell Phones ≠ Self and Other Problems with Big Data Detection and Containment during Epidemics." *Medical Anthropology Quarterly* 32(3): 315–39. https://doi.org/10.1111/maq.12440.
Evans-Pritchard, E. E. 1937. *Witchcraft, Oracles and Magic among the Azande*. Oxford: Oxford University Press.
Fainzang, Sylvie. 1985a. "La 'maison du blanc': la place du dispensaire dans les stratégies thérapeutiques des Bisa du Burkina" [The "white house": The place of the dispensary in the therapeutic strategies of the Bisa of Burkina]. *Sciences Sociales et Santé*: 105–28.
Fainzang, Sylvie. 1985b. "Les Sexes et leurs nombres Sens et fonction du 3 et du 4 dans une société burkinabé" [The sexes and their numbers: Meaning and function of 3 and 4 in Burkinabe society]. *L'Homme* 25(96): 97–109.
Fainzang, Sylvie. 1986. *"L'intérieur des choses": Maladie, divination et reproduction sociale chez les Bisa du Burkina, Connaissance des hommes* ["The inside of things": Illness, divination and social reproduction among the Bisa of Burkina, Knowledge of men]. Paris: L'Harmattan.
Farmer, Paul. 1999. *Infections and Inequalities.The Modern Plagues*. Berkeley: University of California Press.
———. 2006. *AIDS and Accusation: Haiti and the Geography of Blame, Updated with a New Preface*. Berkeley: University of California Press.
Faure, Armelle. 1990. "L'appropriation de l'espace foncier: une étude d'anthropologie sociale en région Bissa (Burkina Faso)" [The appropriation of land space: a study of social anthropology in the Bissa region (Burkina Faso)]. Paris: EHESS.
———. 1996. *Le pays bissa avant le barrage de Bagré. Anthropologie de l'espace rural, Découvertes du Bukina* [The Bissa land around the Bagré dam: Anthropology of rural space, Discoveries of Bukina]. Paris: SÉPIA—A.D.D.B.
Faust, Jörg, Jörn Grävingholt, Sebastian Ziaja. 2015. "Foreign Aid and the Fragile Consensus on State Fragility." *Journal of International Relations and Development* 18(4): 407–27.
Feierman, Steven, and John M. Janzen. 1992. *The Social Basis of Health and Healing in Africa*. Berkeley: University of California Press.

Ferguson, James. 2006. *Global Shadows. Africa in the Neoliberal World Order*. Durham, NC: Duke University Press.

Ferme, Mariane C. 2004. "Deterritorialized Citizenship and the Resonances of the Sierra Leonean State." *Anthropology in the Margins of the State*: 81–115.

Fink, Hans. 2007. "The Conception of Ethics and the Ethical in K. E. Loegstrup's the Ethical Demand." In *Concern for the Other*, 9–28. South Bend, IN: University of Notre Dame Press.

Finkler, Kaja. 1994. "Sacred Healing and Biomedicine Compared." *Medical Anthropology Quarterly* 8(2): 178–97.

Foege, William H., J. Donald Millar, and Donald A Henderson. 1975. "Smallpox Eradication in West and Central Africa." *Bulletin of the World Health Organization* 52(2): 209.

Foley, E. 2009. *Your Pocket Is What Cures You: The Politics of Health in Senegal*. New Brunswick, NJ: Rutgers University Press.

Foucault, Michel. 2007. *Security, Territory, Population: Lectures at the Collège De France, 1977–78*, ed. Michel Senellart, trans. Graham Burchell. Houndmills: Palgrave Macmillan.

———. 2012. *The Birth of the Clinic*. London: Routledge.

Game, Ann. 1997. "Time Unhinged." *Time & Society* 6(2–3): 115–29.

Gamlin, Jennie, Jean Segata, Lina Berrio, Sahra Gibbon, and Francisco Ortega. 2021. "Centring a Critical Medical Anthropology of COVID-19 in Global Health Discourse." *BMJ Global Health* 6(6): e006132.

Gammeltoft, T. M. 2014. *Haunting Images. A Cultural Account of Selective Reproduction in Vietnam*. Berkeley: University of California Press.

Gausset, Q., H. O. Mogensen, W. M. Yameogo, A. Berthe, and B. Konate. 2012. "The Ambivalence of Stigma and the Double-Edged Sword of HIV/AIDS Intervention in Burkina Faso." *Soc Sci Med* 74(7): 1037–44. https://doi.org/10.1016/j.socscimed.2011.11.044.

Gell, Alfred. 1993. *Wrapping in Images: Tattooing in Polynesia*. Oxford: Oxford University Press.

Giddens, Anthony. 1990. *The Consequences of Modernity*. Cambridge: Polity.

Gilson, Lucy, Natasha Palmer, and Helen Schneider. 2005. "Trust and Health Worker Performance: Exploring a Conceptual Framework Using South African Evidence." *Social Science and Medicine* 61(7): 1418–29. https://doi.org/10.1016/j.socscimed.2004.11.062.

Gnawali, D. P., S. Pokhrel, A. Sie, M. Sanon, M. De Allegri, A. Souares, H. Dong, and R. Sauerborn. 2009. "The Effect of Community-Based Health Insurance on the Utilization of Modern Health Care Services: Evidence from Burkina Faso." *Health Policy* 90(2–3): 214–22. https://doi.org/10.1016/j.healthpol.2008.09.015.

Gomez-Temesio, Veronica. 2018. "Outliving Death: Ebola, Zombies, and the Politics of Saving Lives." *American Anthropologist* 120(4): 738–51.

Gottlieb, Alma. 2004. *The Afterlife Is Where We Come From: Infants and Infant Care in West Africa*. Chicago: The University of Chicago Press.

———. 2012. *Under the Kapok Tree: Identity and Difference in Beng Thought*. Chicago: University of Chicago Press.

Gupta, Akhil. 2012. *Red Tape: Bureaucracy, Structural Violence, and Poverty in India*. Durham, NC: Duke University Press.

Haddad, Slim, Adrien Nougtara, and Pierre Fournier. 2006. "Learning from Health System Reforms: Lessons from Burkina Faso." *Tropical Medicine & International Health* 11(12): 1889–97. https://doi.org/10.1111/j.1365-3156.2006.01748.x

Hagberg, Sten. 2019. "Performing Tradition While Doing Politics: A Comparative Study of the Dozos and Koglweogos Self-Defense Movements in Burkina Faso." *African Studies Review* 62(1): 173–93.

Hagberg, Sten, Ludovic Kibora, Sidi Barry, Yacouba Cissao, Siaka Gnessi, Amado Kaboré, Bitou Koné, and Mariatou Zongo. 2019. *Sécurité par le bas: Perceptions et perspectives citoyennes des défis sécurité au Burkina Faso*, Uppsala Papers in Africa Studies, ed. Sten Hagberg. Uppsala: Uppsala University.

Hagberg, Sten, Ludovic Kibora, Sidi Barry, Siaka Gnessi, and Adjara Konkobo. 2018. *"Nothing Will Be as Before!": Anthropological Perspectives on Political Practice and Democratic Culture in a "New Burkina Faso."* Uppsala: Uppsala University.

Hagberg, Sten, Ludovic Kibora, Fatoumata Ouattara, Adjara Konkobo. 2015. "Au cœur de la révolution burkinabè." *Anthropologie & Développement* (42): 199–224.

Hage, Ghassan. 2003. *Searching for Hope in a Shrinking Society*. Sydney: Pluto Press.

———. 2016. "Questions Concerning a Future-Politics." *History and Anthropology* 27(4): 465–67. https://doi.org/10.1080/02757206.2016.1206896.

Handloff, Robert. 1982. "Prayers, Amulets, and Charms: Health and Social Control." *African Studies Review* 25(2–3): 185–94.

Hanks, William F. 1996. "Communicative Practices." *Rethinking Linguistic Relativity* (17): 232.

Hannig, Anita. 2017. *Beyond Surgery: Injury, Healing, and Religion at an Ethiopian Hospital*. Chicago: University of Chicago Press.

Haram, Liv, and C. Bawa Yamba. 2009. *Dealing with Uncertainty in Contemporary African Lives*. Uppsala: Nordiska Afrikainstitutet.

Hewlett, Barry, and Bonnie Hewlett. 2008. *Ebola, Culture, and Politics: The Anthropology of an Emerging Disease*. Belmont, CA: Thomson Wadsworth.

Heyman, Josiah M., and John Symons. 2012. "Borders." In *A Companion to Moral Anthropology*, ed. Didier Fassin, 540–57. Chichester, UK: John Wiley & Sons.

Hinchliffe, Steve, and Kim J. Ward. 2014. "Geographies of Folded Life: How Immunity Reframes Biosecurity." *Geoforum* 53: 136–44. https://doi.org/10.1016/j.geoforum.2014.03.002.

Hodgson, Dorothy L. 2017. "Africa from the Margins." *African Studies Review* 60(2): 37–49.

Holden, Pat, and Jenny Littlewood. 2015. *Anthropology and Nursing*. London: Routledge.

Holmes, Seth. 2013. *Fresh Fruit, Broken Bodies: Migrant Farmworkers in the United States*, vol. 27. Berkeley: University of California Press.

Huskey, Rebecca Kathleen. 2009. *Paul Ricœur on Hope: Expecting the Good*, vol. 6. Frankfurt: Peter Lang.

Hutchinson, Eleanor, Clare Chandler, Siân Clarke, Sham Lal, Pascal Magnussen, Miriam Kayendeke, Christine Nabirye, James Kizito, and Anthony Mbonye. 2015. "'It Puts Life in Us and We Feel Big': Shifts in the Local Health Care System during the Introduction of Rapid Diagnostic Tests for Malaria into Drug Shops in Uganda." *Critical Public Health* 25(1): 48–62.

Hutchinson, Eleanor, Susan Nayiga, Christine Nabirye, Lilian Taaka, and Sarah G. Staedke. 2018. "Data Value and Care Value in the Practice of Health Systems: A Case Study in Uganda." *Social Science & Medicine* 211: 123–10.

Hutchinson, Eleanor, Hugh Reyburn, Eleanor Hamlyn, Katie Long, Judith Meta, Hilda Mbakilwa, and Clare Chandler. 2017. "Bringing the State into the Clinic? Incorporating the Rapid Diagnostic Test for Malaria into Routine Practice in Tanzanian Primary Healthcare Facilities." *Global Public Health* 12(9): 1077–91.

Hynes, William J. 1993. "Mapping the Characteristics of Mythic Tricksters: A Heuristic Guide." *Mythical Trickster Figures: Contours, Contexts, and Criticisms*, ed. William J. Hynes and William G. Doty, 33–45. Tuscaloosa: The University of Alabama Press.

Hänsch, Valerie, Lena Kroeker, and Silke Oldenburg. 2017. "Uncertain Future(s)." *TSANTSA–Journal of the Swiss Anthropological Association* 22: 4–17.

ICF, INSD. 2022. "Enquête Démographique et de Santé." Ouagadougou: INSD and ICF.

Imperato, Pascal James. 1977. *African Folk Medicine: Practices and Beliefs of the Bambara and Other Peoples*. Baltimore, MD: York Press.

Inda, Jonathan Xavier, and Renato Rosaldo. 2002. *The Anthropology of Globalization : A Reader, Blackwell Readers in Anthropology*. Malden, MA: Blackwell Publishers.

INSD. 2012. *Enquête Démographique et de Santé et à Indicateurs Multiples du Burkina Faso 2010*. Calverton, MD: INSD and ICF International.

INSD 2021. *The DHS Program*. Rockville, MD: ICF. *Burkina Faso Enquête Démographique et de Santé 2021* (French). Rockville, MD: INSD/DHS.

INSD and Macro International Inc. 2000. *Enquête Démographiqueet de Santé, Burkina Faso 1998–1999*. Calverton, MD: Macro International Inc.

Jackson, Michael. 1998. *Minima Ethnographica: Intersubjectivity and the Anthropological Project*. Chicago: University of Chicago Press.

Janzen, J. 1978. *The Quest for Therapy: Medical Pluralism in Lower Zaire*. Berkeley: University of California Press.

Jerven, Morten. 2008. "African Economic Growth Reconsidered: Measurement and Performance in East-Central Africa, 1965–1995." Ph.D. dissertation. London: London School of Economics and Political Science (University of London).

———. 2013. *Poor Numbers: How We Are Misled by African Development Statistics and What to Do about It*. Ithaca, NY: Cornell University Press.

Kaboré, Saidou, Philippe Cecchi, Thomas Mosser, Mylène Toubiana, Oumar Traoré, Aboubakar S. Ouattara, Alfred S. Traoré, Nicolas Barro, Rita R. Colwell, and Patrick Monfort. 2018. "Occurrence of Vibrio Cholerae in Water Reservoirs of Burkina Faso." *Research in Microbiology* 169(1): 1–10.

Kagoné, Moubassira, Maurice Yé, Eric Nébié, Ali Sie, Anja Schoeps, Heiko Becher, Olaf Muller, and Ane Baerent Fisker. 2017. "Vaccination Coverage and Factors Associated with Adherence to the Vaccination Schedule in Young Children of a Rural Area in Burkina Faso." *Global Health Action* 10(1): 1399749.

Kandel, Nirmal, Stella Chungong, Abbas Omaar, and Jun Xing. 2020. "Health Security Capacities in the Context of COVID-19 Outbreak: An Analysis of International Health Regulations Annual Report Data from 182 Countries." *The Lancet* 395(10229): 1047–53.

Kaschula, Russell H. 1999. "Imbongi and Griot: Toward a Comparative Analysis of Oral Poetics in Southern and West Africa." *Journal of African Cultural Studies* 12(1): 55–76.

Katahoire, Anne, Flemming Scheutz, Svend Sabroe, and S. Reynolds Whyte. 2004. "The Importance of Maternal Schooling for Child Morbidity and Mortality and Maternal Health Behavior in Southeastern Uganda." *Journal of Health & Population in Developing Countries* 6(1): 12.

Kearney, Richard. 1996. *Paul Ricoeur: The Hermeneutics of Action*. London: Sage.

Keja, K., C. Chan, G. Hayden, and R. H. Henderson. 1988. "Expanded Programme on Immunization." *World Health Statistics Quarterly—Rapport trimestriel de statistiques sanitaires mondiales* 41(2): 59–63.

Kelly, Ann H., Frédéric Keck, and Christos Lynteris. 2019. *The Anthropology of Epidemics*. London: Routledge.

Kessler, S., F. Falaha, G. L. Gonidec, and D. Parker. 1986. *Lessons Learned: Rapid Assessment: Vaccination Commando Burkina Faso*. New York: UNICEF.

Kingori, Patricia 2013. "Experiencing Everyday Ethics in Context: Frontline Data Collectors Perspectives and Practices of Bioethics." *Social Science & Medicine* 98: 361–70.

Kleinman, Arthur. 1978. "Concepts and a Model for the Comparison of Medical Systems as Cultural Systems." *Social Science & Medicine. Part B: Medical Anthropology* 12: 85–93.

———. 1980. *Patients and Healers in the Context of Culture*. Berkeley: University of California Press.

Kleist, Nauja, and Jesper Bjarnesen. 2019. "Migration Infrastructures in West Africa and Beyond." *Miasa Working Paper* (3): 1–23.

Kleist, Nauja, and Stef Jansen. 2016. "Introduction: Hope over Time—Crisis, Immobility and Future-Making." *History and Anthropology* 27(4): 373–392. https://doi.org/10.1080/02757206.2016.1207636.

Korbeogo, Gabin. 2013. *Pouvoir et accès aux ressources naturelles au Burkina Faso: La topographie du pouvoir*. Paris: L'Harmattan.

Koulidiati, Jean-Louis, Manuela De Allegri, Aurelia Souares, Samiratou Ouedraogo, Hervé Hien, Paul Jacob Robyn, and Stephan Brenner. 2018. "Factors Associated with Effective Coverage of Child Health Services in Burkina Faso." *Tropical Medicine & International Health* 23(11): 1188–99.

Kruk, Margaret E., Stephanie Kujawski, Godfrey Mbaruku, Kate Ramsey, Wema Moyo, and Lynn P. Freedman. 2018. "Disrespectful and Abusive Treatment during Facility Delivery in Tanzania: A Facility and Community Survey." *Health Policy and Planning*: e26-e33.

Lahuec, Jean-Paul, and Jean-Yves Marchal. 1979. *La mobilité du peuplement Bissa et Mossi*. [The mobility of the Bissa and Mossi populations] Paris: l'orstom.

Lakoff, Andrew. 2017. *Unprepared: Global Health in a Time of Emergency*. Berkeley: University of California Press.

Lambek, Michael. 2010. *Ordinary Ethics: Anthropology, Language, and Action*. New York: Fordham University Press.

Langwick, Stacey A. 2007. "Devils, Parasites, and Fierce Needles: Healing and the Politics of Translation in Southern Tanzania." *Science, Technology, Human Values* 32(1): 88–117.

Larkan, Fiona, Caroline Ryan, and Sebastian Kevany. 2015. "The Geopolitics of Ebola and Global Health Security: Why Anthropology Matters." *Irish Journal of Anthropology* 2015(18): 1.

Laugier, Sandra 2015. "The Ethics of Care as a Politics of the Ordinary." *New Literary History* 46(2): 217–40.

Law, John. 2002. *Aircraft Stories*. Durham, NC: Duke University Press.

Levi-Strauss, Claude. 1963. *Structural Anthropology*. New York: S. L. Basic Books.

Livingston, Julie. 2012. *Improvising Medicine: An African Oncology Ward in an Emerging Cancer Epidemic*. Durham, NC: Duke University Press.

Long, Debbi, Cynthia Hunter, and Sjaak Van der Geest. 2008. "When the Field Is a Ward or a Clinic: Hospital Ethnography." *Anthropology & Medicine* 15(2): 71–78.

Lucht, Hans. 2011. *Darkness before Daybreak: African Migrants Living on the Margins in Southern Italy Today*. Berkeley: University of California Press.

Lynteris, Christos. 2014. "Introduction: The Time of Epidemics." *The Cambridge Journal of Anthropology* 32(1): 24–31.

Lynteris, Christos, and Branwyn Poleykett. 2018. "The Anthropology of Epidemic Control: Technologies and Materialities." *Medical Anthropology* 37(6): 433–41. https://doi.org/10.1080/01459740.2018.1484740.

Løgstrup, Knud Ejler. 1991. *Den etiske fordring*. Viborg: Gyldendal.

———. 1997. *The Ethical Demand*. South Bend, IN: University of Notre Dame Pess.

MacGregor, Hayley, Melissa Leach, Grace Akello, Lawrence Sao Babawo, Moses Baluku, Alice Desclaux, Catherine Grant, Foday Kamara, Fred Martineau, and Esther Yei Mokuwa. 2022. "Negotiating Intersecting Precarities: COVID-19, Pandemic Preparedness and Response in Africa." *Medical Anthropology* 41(1): 19–33.

MacLean, Lauren M. J. 2011. "State Retrenchment and the Exercise of Citizenship in Africa." *Comparative Political Studies* 44(9): 1238–66.

Manderson, Lenore, and Susan Levine. 2021. "Militarising the Pandemic: Lockdown in South Africa." In *Viral Loads: Anthropologies of Urgency in the*

Time of COVID-19, ed. Lenore Manderson, Nancy J. Burke, Ayo Wahlberg, 47–66. London: UCL Press.
Manderson, Lenore, Nancy J. Burke, and Ayo Wahlberg. 2021. *Viral Loads: Anthropologies of urgency in the time of COVID-19*. London UCL Press,
Manderson, Lenore and Carolyn Smith-Morris. "Introduction. Chronicity and the Experience of Illness," in *Chronic Conditions, Fluid States, Rutgers Studies in Medical Anthropology*, eds Lenore Manderson, Muhana Utami, Carolyn Smith-Morris, Marcia Inhorn, Arthur Kleinman, Rachel Hall-Clifford, Dennis Wiedman, Byron Good, Carla Manchira, and Nida Hasanat, 1–18. New Brunswick, NJ: Rutgers University Press.
Manderson, Lenore, Muhana Utami, Carolyn Smith-Morris, Marcia Inhorn, Arthur Kleinman, Rachel Hall-Clifford, Dennis Wiedman, Byron Good, Carla Manchira, and Nida Hasanat. 2010. *Chronic Conditions, Fluid States : Chronicity and the Anthropology of Illness*. New Brunswick, NJ, UNITED STATES: Rutgers University Press.
Manderson, Lenore, and Narelle Warren. 2016. "'Just One Thing after Another': Recursive Cascades and Chronic Conditions." *Medical Anthropology Quarterly* 30(4): 479–97.
Maradze, Takudzwa C., Smartson P. Nyoni, and Thabani Nyoni. 2021. "Modelling and Forecasting Child Immunization against Measles Disease in Burkina Faso Using Artificial Neural Networks (ANN)." *International Research Journal of Innovations in Engineering and Technology* 5(3): 487.
Mason, Katherine. 2016. *Infectious Change: Reinventing Chinese Public Health after an Epidemic*. Stanford, CA: Stanford University Press.
Masquelier, Adeline Marie. 2001. "Behind the Dispensary's Prosperous Façade: Imagining the State in Rural Niger." *Public Culture* 13(2): 267–91.
Mauss, Marcel. 2001. *A General Theory of Magic*. London: Psychology Press.
McKay, Ramah. 2017. *Medicine in the Meantime: the Work of Care in Mozambique*. Durham, NC: Duke University Press.
McMillan, Della E. 1995. *Sahel Visions: Planned Settlement and River Blindness Control in Burkina Faso*. Tucson: University of Arizona Press.
Melberg, Andrea, Abdoulaye Hama Diallo, Ana Lorena Ruano, Thorkild Tylleskär, and Karen Marie Moland. 2016. "Reflections on the Unintended Consequences of the Promotion of Institutional Pregnancy and Birth Care in Burkina Faso." *PloS one* 11(6): e0156503.
Melberg, Andrea, Abdoulaye Hama Diallo, Thorkild Tylleskär, and Karen Marie Moland. 2016. "'We Saw She Was in Danger, but Couldn't Do Anything': Missed Opportunities and Health Worker Disempowerment during Birth Care in Rural Burkina Faso." *BMC Pregnancy and Childbirth* 16(1): 292.
Mengel, Martin A., Isabelle Delrieu, Leonard Heyerdahl, and Bradford D. Gessner. 2014. "Cholera Outbreaks in Africa." *Cholera Outbreaks*: 117–44.
Merry, Sally Engle. 2011. "Measuring the World." *Current Anthropology* 52(S3): S83–S95. https://doi.org/10.1086/657241.
Meunier, Aude. 1999. *Système de soins au Burkina Faso: Le paradoxe sanitaire*. Paris: L'Harmattan.

Mikal, Jude, Kathryn Grace, Jack DeWaard, Molly Brown, and Gabriel Sangli. 2020. "Domestic Migration and Mobile Phones: A Qualitative Case Study Focused on Recent Migrants to Ouagadougou, Burkina Faso." *PloS one* 15(8): e0236248.

Millar, Kathleen. 2014. "The Precarious Present: Wageless Labor and Disrupted Life in Rio De Janeiro, Brazil." *Cultural Anthropology* 29(1): 32–53.

Ministère de la Santé, Burkina Faso. 2011. *Plan National de Developpement Sanitaire 2011–2020*. Ouagadougou: Ministère de la Santé.

Ministère de la Santé, Burkina Faso. 2017. *Directives Nationales De Prise En Charge Du Paludisme*. Ouagadougou: Ministère de la Santé.

Ministère de la Santé, Burkina Faso. 2018. *Bulletin D'épidèmiologie Et D'information Sanitaire. Deuxième Triemstre 2018*. Ouagadougou: Ministère de la Santé.

Ministère de la Santé, Burkina Faso. 2019. *Annuaire Statistique De La Santé 2018*, ed. Conseil National de la Statistique CNS. Ouagadougou: Ministère de la Santé.

Ministère de la Santé, Burkina Faso. 2020. *Plan De Preparation Et De Riposte À L'épidemie De COVID-19 Au Burkina Faso*. Revisé. Ouagadougou: Ministère de la Santé.

Ministère de la Santé, Burkina Faso. 2022. *Annuaire Statistique 2021*, ed. Direction générale des études et des statistiques sectorielles. Ouagadougou: Ministère de la Santé.

Mitchell, Matthew I. 2012. "Migration, Citizenship and Autochthony: Strategies and Challenges for State-Building in Côte d'Ivoire." *Journal of Contemporary African Studies* 30(2): 267–87.

Mkhwanazi, Nolwazi. 2016. "Medical Anthropology in Africa: The Trouble with a Single Story." *Medical Anthropology* 35(2): 193–202.

Mogensen, Hanne O. 2005. "Finding a Path through the Health Unit: Practical Experience of Ugandan Patients." *Medical Anthropology* 24(3): 209–36. https://doi.org/10.1080/01459740500182659.

Mol, Annemarie. 2002. *The Body Mulitiple: Ontology in Medical Practice, Science and Cultural Theory*. Durham, NC: Duke University Press.

———. 2008. *The Logic of Care: Health and the Problem of Patient Choice*. London: Routledge.

Müller, Olaf, Corneille Traoré, Heiko Becher, and Bocar Kouyaté. 2003. "Malaria Morbidity, Treatment-Seeking Behaviour, and Mortality in a Cohort of Young Children in Rural Burkina Faso." *Tropical Medicine and International Health* 8(4): 290–96.

Nguyen, Vinh-Kim. 2010. *The Republic of Therapy: Triage and Sovereignty in West Africa's Time of AIDS*. Durham, NC: Duke University Press.

Nyamweya, Nancy Nyasuguta, Peter Yekka, Ronny Drasi Mubutu, Keneth Iceland Kasozi, and Jane Muhindo. 2017. "Staff Absenteeism in Public Health Facilities of Uganda: A Study in Bushenyi District on Contributing Factors." *Open Journal of Nursing* 7(10): 1115.

Obadare, Ebenezer, and Wale Adebanwi. 2010. "Introduction: Excess and Abjection in the Study of the African State." In *Encountering the Nigerian State*, 1–28. New York: Palgrave Macmillan.

OECD. 2010. *The State's Legitimacy in Fragile Situations: Unpacking Complexity*. Paris: OECD.

Okri, Ben. (1991) 1993. *The Famished Road*. New York: Anchor.

Olivier de Sardan, Jean-Pierre. 2008. "State Bureaucracy and Governance in Francophone West Africa: An Empirical Diagnosis and Historical Perspective." In *The Governance of Daily Life in Africa*, 39–71. Leiden: Brill.

———. 2015. "Practical Norms: Informal Regulations within Public Bureaucracies (in Africa and Beyond)." In *Real Governance and Practical Norms in Sub-Saharan Africa: The Game of the Rules*, ed. Tom De Herdt and Jean-Pierre Olivier de Sardan, 19–62. Abingdon: Routledge.

Olsen, William C., and Carolyn Sargent. 2017. *African Medical Pluralism*. Bloomington: Indiana University Press.

Østergaard, L. R. 2015. "Maternal Healthcare in Context: A Qualitative Study of Women's Tactics to Improve Their Experience of Public Healthcare in Rural Burkina Faso." *Social Science & Medicine* 147: 98–104. https://doi.org/10.1016/j.socscimed.2015.10.062.

Østergaard, Lise Rosendal, Pia Juul Bjertrup, and Helle Samuelsen. 2016. "'Children Get Sick All the Time': A Qualitative Study of Socio-Cultural and Health System Factors Contributing to Recurrent Child Illnesses in Rural Burkina Faso." *BMC Public Health* 16(1): 384.

Ouédraogo, Mady, David Tiga Kangoye, Sékou Samadoulougou, Toussaint Rouamba, Philippe Donnen, and Fati Kirakoya-Samadoulougou. 2020. "Malaria Case Fatality Rate among Children under Five in Burkina Faso: An Assessment of the Spatiotemporal trends following the Implementation of Control Programs." *International Journal of Environmental Research and Public Health* 17(6): 1840.

Ouédraogo, Nobila, Moubassira Kagoné, Ali Sié, Heiko Becher, and Olaf Müller. 2013. "Immunization Coverage in Young Children: A Study Nested into a Health and Demographic Surveillance System in Burkina Faso." *Journal of Tropical Pediatrics* 59(3): 187–94. https://doi.org/10.1093/tropej/fms075.

Oxford English Dictionary. 2008. "Ambiguity." In *Oxford English Dictionary*. Oxford: Oxford University Press.

Pale, Siébou, Sibiri Jean-Baptiste Taonda, Boniface Bougouma, and Stephen C. Mason. 2010. "Sorghum Malt and Traditional Beer (Dolo) Quality Assessment in Burkina Faso." *Ecology of Food and Nutrition* 49(2): 129–41.

Pare Toe, Lea, and Helle Samuelsen. 2020. "Balancing Professional Autonomy and Authority at the Margins of a Fragile State: Front-Line Health Workers' Experiences in Burkina Faso." *Global Public Health* 16(7): 1099–1110.

Parker, Melissa, Hayley MacGregor, and Grace Akello. 2020. "COVID-19, Public Authority and Enforcement." *Medical Anthropology* 39(8): 666–70.

Pelton, Robert D. 1989. *The Trickster in West Africa: A Study of Mythic Irony and Sacred Delight*. Berkeley: University of California Press.

Petryna, Adriana. 2002. *Life Exposed: Biological Citizens after Chernobyl*. Princeton, NJ: Princeton University Press.

Petryna, Adriana. 2013a. *Life Exposed: Biological Citizens after Chernobyl*, revised ed. Princeton, NJ: Princeton University Press.

Petryna, Adriana 2013b. "The Right of Recovery." *Current Anthropology* 54(S7): S67–S76.

Pierre Ilboudo, Tegawende, Yiing-Jenq Chou, and Nicole Huang. 2012. "Compliance with Referral for Curative Care in Rural Burkina Faso." *Health Policy and Planning* 27(3): 256–64.

Porter, Theodore M. 1996. *Trust in Numbers: The Pursuit of Objectivity in Science and Public Life*. Princeton, NJ: Princeton University Press.

Prince, Ruth, and Rebecca Marsland. 2014. *Making and Unmaking Public Health in Africa: Ethnographic and Historical Perspectives, Cambridge Center of African Studies*. Athens: Ohio University Press.

Rasmussen, Stine Loft. 2017. "Practices of Disease Surveillance and Response in Burkina Faso." International Conference on Social Implications of Computers in Developing Countries, 333–44. May 2017, Yogyakarta, Indonesia.

Rasmussen, Stine Loft, and Sundeep Sahay. 2022. "Multiplicity and Temporality of Rationality: Constructing Information for Meningitis Surveillance and Response in Burkina Faso." *The Information Society* 38(1): 51–76.

REN-LAC. 2018. *Etude sur les presomptions de corruption et pratiques assimilees dans le systeme et les services de santé au Burkina Faso*. [Study on the presumptions of corruption and similar practices in the health system and services in Burkina Faso] Ouagadougou: Réseau National de Lutte Anti-corruption.

Ribera, Joan Muela, and Susanna Hausmann Muela. 2011. "The Straw that Breaks the Camel's Back: Redirecting Health Seeking Behavior Studies on Malaria and Vulnerability." *Medical Anthropology Quarterly* 25(1): 103–21.

Ricoeur, Paul. 1986. *Fallible Man*, vol. 1. New York: Fordham Univ Press.

———. 1994. *Oneself as Another*. Chicago: University of Chicago Press.

———. 1996. "Fragility and Responsibility." In *Paul Ricoeur. The Hermeneutics of Action*, ed. Richard Kearney, 15–22. London: Sage Publications.

Ricoeur, Paul, and Richard Kearney. 1996. *Paul Ricoeur: The Hermeneutics of Action*, vol. 2. London: Sage Publications.

Ridde, Valéry, Ludovic Queuille, Nicole Atchessi, Omar Samb, Rolf Heinmüller, and Slim Haddad. 2013. "The Evaluation of an Experiment in Healthcare User Fees Exemption for Vulnerable Groups in Burkina Faso." *Field Actions Science Reports: The Journal of Field Actions* (Special Issue 8).

Riedel, Stefan. 2005. "Edward Jenner and the History of Smallpox and Vaccination." *Baylor University Medical Center Proceedings* 18(1): 21–25.

Rifkin, Susan B. 2018. "Alma Ata after 40 Years: Primary Health Care and Health for All-from Consensus to Complexity." *BMJ Global Health* 3(Suppl 3): e001188–e001188. https://doi.org/10.1136/bmjgh-2018-001188.

Robinson, Fiona. 1997. "Globalizing Care: Ethics, Feminist Theory, and International Relations." *Alternatives* 22(1): 113–33.

Rubin, Arnold. 1988. *Marks of Civilization, Artistic Transformations of the Human Body*, ed. Arnold Rubin. Los Angeles: Museum of Cultural History, University of California.

Ruckenstein, Minna, and Natasha Dow Schüll. 2017. "The Datafication of Health." *Annual Review of Anthropology* 46: 261–78.

Samuelsen, Helle., Britt. P. Tersbol, and Selimani. S. Mbuyita. 2013. "Do Health Systems Delay the Treatment of Poor Children? A Qualitative Study of Child Deaths in Rural Tanzania." *BMC Health Services Research* 13: 67. https://doi.org/10.1186/1472-6963-13-67.

Samuelsen, Helle. 1998. "Åndebørn." *Tidsskriftet Antropologi* 38: 95–105.

———. 1999. "The Topology of Illness Transmission: Localizing Processes among Bissa in Burkina Faso." Ph.D dissertation. Copenhagen: University of Copenhagen.

———. 2001. "Infusions of Health: The Popularity of Vaccinations among Bissa in Burkina Faso." *Anthropology & Medicine* 8(2–3): 163–75.

———. 2004a. "Illness Transmission and Proximity: Local Theories of Causation among the Bissa in Burkina Faso." *Medical Anthropology* 23(2): 89–112. https://doi.org/10.1080/01459740490448885.

———. 2004b. "Therapeutic Itineraries: The Medical Field in Rural Burkina Faso." *Anthropology & Medicine* 11(1): 27–41.

———. 2016. "Health Care Systems." In *International Encyclopedia of Anthropology*, ed. Hilary Callan. Hoboken, NJ: Wiley Blackwell.

———. 2022. "Fragile Relationships: Elusive Encounters with Public Services in Rural Burkina Faso." In *Everyday State and Democracy in Africa: Ethnographic Encounters*, ed. Wale Adebanwi, 384–402. Athens: Ohio University Press.

Samuelsen, Helle, Ole Norgaard, and Lise Rosendal Ostergaard. 2012. "Social and Cultural Aspects of HIV and AIDS in West Africa: A Narrative Review of Qualitative Research." *SAHARA: Journal of Social Aspects of HIV/AIDS Research Alliance / SAHARA, Human Sciences Research Council* 9(2): 64–73.

Samuelsen, Helle, and Vibeke Steffen. 2004. "The Relevance of Foucault and Bourdieu for Medical Anthropology: Exploring New Sites." *Anthropology & Medicine* 11(1): 3–10.

Samuelsen, Helle, and Lea Paré Toé. 2021. "Covid-19 Temporalities: Ruptures of Everyday Life in Urban Burkina Faso." *Medicine Anthropology Theory* 8(1): 1–21.

Sargent, Carolyn Fishel. 1989. "Maternity, Medicine, and Power." In *Maternity, Medicine, and Power*. Berkeley: University of California Press.

Sarrassat, S., N. Meda, H. Badolo, M. Ouedraogo, H. Somé, and S. Cousens. 2019. "Distance to Care, Care Seeking and Child Mortality in Rural Burkina Faso: Findings from a Population-Based Cross-Sectional Survey." *Tropical Medicine & International Health* 24(1): 31–42.

Saul, Mahir 1981. "Beer, Sorghum and Women: Production for the Market in Rural Upper Volta." *Africa* 51(3): 746–64.

Savage, Roger W. H. 2013. "Fragile Identities, Capable Selves." *Études Ricoeuriennes/Ricoeur Studies* 4(2): 64–78.

Schapendonk, Joris, Matthieu Bolay, and Janine Dahinden. 2020. "The Conceptual Limits of the 'Migration Journey': De-Exceptionalising Mobility in the Context of West African Trajectories." *Journal of Ethnic and Migration Studies* 47(14): 3243–59. https://doi.org/10.1080/1369183X.2020.1804191.

Scheper-Hughes, Nancy. 2014. "Family Life as Bricolage-Reflections on Intimacy and Attachment in Death without Weeping." In *Different Faces of*

Attachment: Cultural Variations on a Universal Human Need, 230–60. New York: Cambridge University Press.

Scherz, China. 2018. "Stuck in the Clinic: Vernacular Healing and Medical Anthropology in Contemporary Sub-Saharan Africa." *Medical Anthropology Quarterly* 32(4): 539–55.

Schieffelin, John S., Jeffrey G. Shaffer, Augustine Goba, Michael Gbakie, Stephen K. Gire, Andres Colubri, Rachel S.G. Sealfon, Lansana Kanneh, Alex Moigboi, Mambu Momoh, et al. 2014. "Clinical Illness and Outcomes in Patients with Ebola in Sierra Leone." *New England Journal of Medicine* 371(22): 2092–100. https://doi.org/10.1056/NEJMoa1411680.

Schildkrout, Enid. 2004. "Inscribing the Body." *Annual Review of Anthropology* 33: 319–44.

Schaafsma, Petruschka 2014. "Philosophical Anthropology against Objectification: Reconsidering Ricoeur's Fallible Man." *International Journal of Philosophy & Theology* 75(2): 152–68.

Scott, James C. 1998. *Seeing like a State: How Certain Schemes to Improve the Human Condition Have Failed*. New Haven, CT: Yale University Press.

Sharma, Aradhana, and Akhil Gupta. 2006. "Introduction: Rethinking Theories of the State in an Age of Globalization." In *The Anthropology of the State: A Reader*, ed. Aradhana Sharma and Akhil Gupta. Malden, MA: Blackwell Publishing.

Sjørslev, Inger. 2015. *Sandhed & genre: Videnskabsteori i antropologi og kulturanalyse* [Truth & genre: Theory of science in anthropology and cultural analysis]. Fredriksberg, Denmark: Samfundslitteratur.

Soeters, Heidi M., Alpha Oumar Diallo, Brice W. Bicaba, Goumbi Kadadé, Assétou Y. Dembélé, Mahamat A. Acyl, Christelle Nikiema, Adodo Yao Sadji, Alain N. Poy, and Clement Lingani. 2019. "Bacterial Meningitis Epidemiology in Five Countries in the Meningitis Belt of Sub-Saharan Africa, 2015–2017." *The Journal of Infectious Diseases* 220(Supplement_4): S165–S174.

Sombié, Issa, David O. S. Ilboudo, André Kamba Soubeiga, and Helle Samuelsen. 2017. "Comprendre l'influence des facteurs contextuels sur la participation communautaire à la santé: une étude de cas dans le district sanitaire de Tenkodogo, au Burkina Faso" [Understanding the influence of contextual factors on community participation in health: A case study in the health district of Tenkodogo, Burkina Faso] *Global Health Promotion* 24(3): 87–95.

Stewart, Alexandra J., and Phillip M. Devlin. 2006. "The History of the Smallpox Vaccine." *Journal of Infection* 52(5): 329–34.

Strathern, Andrew. 1996. *Body Thoughts*. Ann Arbor: University of Michigan Press.

Street, Alice. 2012. "Seen by the State: Bureaucracy, Visibility and Governmentality in a Papua New Guinean Hospital." *The Australian Journal of Anthropology* 23(1): 1–21. https://doi.org/10.1111/j.1757-6547.2012.00164.x.

———. 2014. *Biomedicine in an Unstable Place: Infrastructure and Personhood in a Papua New Guinean Hospital*. Durham, NC: Duke University Press.

Strong, Adrienne E. 2020. *Documenting Death: Maternal Mortality and the Ethics of Care in Tanzania*. Berkeley: University of California Press.

Team, Victoria, and Lenore Manderson. 2020. "How COVID-19 Reveals Structures of Vulnerability." *Medical Anthropology* 39(8): 671–74.
Tichenor, Marlee. 2017. "Data Performativity, Performing Health Work: Malaria and Labor in Senegal." *Medical Anthropology* 36(5): 436–48.
Timmermans, Stefan, and Steven Epstein. 2010. "A World of Standards but Not a Standard World: Toward a Sociology of Standards and Standardization." *Annual Review of Sociology*: 69–89. https://doi.org/10.1146/annurev.soc.012809.102629.
Torres, R. M. 2015. "Gendered Costs to the 'Left Behind': A Challenge to the Migration and Development Nexus." In *The Routledge Handbook of Gender and Development*, ed. Anne Coles, Leslie Gray, and Janet Momsen. Abingdon: Routledge.
Trentmann, Frank. 2020. "Disruption Is Normal: Blackouts, Breakdowns and the Elasticity of Everyday Life." In *Time, Consumption and Everyday Life*, ed. Elizabeth Shove, Frank Trentmann, and Richard Wilk, 67–84. Abingdon: Routledge.
Turner, Simon. 2015. "'We Wait for Miracles': Ideas of Hope and Future among Clandestine Burundian Refugees in Nairobi." In *Ethnographies of Uncertainty in Africa*, ed. Elizabeth Cooper and David Pratten, 173–91. Houndmills: Palgrave Macmillan.
Turner, Victor. 1967. *The Forest of Symbols: Aspects of Ndembu Ritual*, vol. 101. Ithaca, NY: Cornell University Press.
UNDP. 2019. *Independent Country Programme Evaluation: Burkina Faso*. New York: UNDP.
UNICEF. 1985. "Vaccination Commando In Burkina Faso: The Spearhead for Accelerated EPI and PHC." *Assignment Children* (6): 301–27.
———. 1998. *State of the World's Children Report*. New York: UNICEF.
———. 2019. *The State of the World's Children*. New York: UNICEF.
Van Beek, Walter E. A., and Pieteke M. Banga. 2002. "The Dogon and Their Trees." In *Bush Base, Forest Farm*, ed. Elisabeth Croll and David Parkin, 69–87. London: Routledge.
Van der Geest, Sjaak, and Kaja Finkler. 2004. "Hospital Ethnography: Introduction." *Social Science & Medicine* 59(10): 1995–2001.
Van der Geest, Sjaak, and Susan Reynolds Whyte, eds. 1988. *The Context of Medicines in Developing Countries*. Amsterdam: Het Spinhuis.
Van der Geest, Sjaak, Susan Reynolds Whyte, and Anita Hardon. 1996. "The Anthropology of Pharmaceuticals: A Biographical Approach." *Annual Review of Anthropology* 25(1): 153–78.
Van Gennep, Arnold. 2013. *The Rites of Passage*. London: Routledge.
Van Nistelrooij, Inge, Petruschka Schaafsma, and Joan C. Tronto. 2014. "Ricoeur and the Ethics of Care." *Medicine, Health Care and Philosophy* 17: 485–91.
Van Nistelrooy, Inge. 2014. "Self-Sacrifice and Self-Affirmation Within Care-Giving." *Medicine, Health Care and Philosophy* 17(4): 519–28.
Vaughan, Megan. 2007. "Scarification in Africa." *Cultural and Social History* 4(3): 385–400. https://doi.org/10.2752/147800407X219269.

Venkatesan, Priya. 2022. "Global Polio Eradication Set Back by COVID-19 Pandemic." *The Lancet Microbe* 3(3): e172.

Vigh, Henrik. 2008. "Crisis and Chronicity: Anthropological Perspectives on Continuous Conflict and Decline." *Ethnos* 73(1): 5–24. https://doi.org/10.1080/00141840801927509.

———. 2009. "Wayward Migration: on Imagined Futures and Technological Voids." *Ethnos* 74(1): 91–109.

———. 2011. "Vigilance: On Conflict, Social Invisibility, and Negative Potentiality." *Social Analysis* 55(3): 93–114.

———. 2017. "Caring through Crime: Ethical Ambivalence and the Cocaine Trade in Bissau." *Africa* 87(3): 479–95.

von Maydell, Hans-Jürgen. 1986. *Trees and Shrubs of the Sahel, Their Characteristics and Uses*. Eschborn: GTZ.

Wahlberg, Ayo, and Tine M Gammeltoft. 2018. *Selective Reproduction in the 21st Century*. Cham: Springer International Publishing.

Watts, Sheldon. 1997. *Epidemics and History: Disease Power and Imperialism*. New Haven, CT: Yale University Press.

Weber, Max. 1978. *Economy and Society: An Outline of Interpretive Sociology*, vol. 1. Berkeley: University of California Press.

WEF. 2016. *The Global Risk Report*, 11th edn. Geneva: World Economic Forum.

Wendland, Claire. 2016. "Estimating Death: A Close Reading of Maternal Mortality Metrics in Malawi." In *Metrics: What Counts in Global Health*, ed. Vincanne Adams, 57–81. Durham, NC: Duke University Press.

———. 2010. *A Heart for the Work: Journeys through an African Medical School*. Chicago: University of Chicago Press.

WHO. 2011. *The Abuja Declaration: Ten Years On*. Geneva: World Health Organization.

———. 2015. *World Malaria Report*. Geneva: World Health Organization

———. 2018. *Managing Epidemics: Key Facts about Major Deadly Diseases*. Geneva: World Health Organization.

Whyte, Susan Reynolds. 1997. *Questioning Misfortune : The Pragmatics of Uncertainty in Eastern Uganda*. Cambridge: Cambridge University Press.

———. 2005. "Uncertain Undertakings: Practicing Health Care in the Subjunctive Mood." In *Managing Uncertainty: Ethnographic Studies of Illness, Risk and the Struggle for Control*, ed. Vibeke Steffen, Richard Jenkins, and Hanne Jessen, 245–64. Copenhagen: Museum Tusculanum Press.

———. 2009. "Epilogue." In *Dealing with Uncertainties in Contemporariy African Lives*, ed. Liv Haram and Bawa Yamba, 213–15. Stockholm: Nordiska Afrika Institutet.

———, ed. 2014. *Second Chances. Surviving AIDS in Uganda*. Durham, NC: Duke University Press.

Whyte, Susan Reynolds, Sjaak Van der Geest, and Anita Hardon. 2002. *Social Lives of Medicines*. Cambridge: Cambridge University Press.

Whyte, Susan Reynolds, Michael Whyte, Lotte Meinert, and Jennipher Twebaze. 2013. "Therapeutic Clientship: Belonging in Uganda's Projectified Landscape of AIDS Care." In *When People Come First: Critical Studies in

Global Health, ed. João Biehl and Adriana Petryna. Princeton, NJ: Princeton University Press.

Wilkinson, Iain, and Arthur Kleinman. 2016. *A Passion for Society: How We Think about Human Suffering, California Series in Public Anthropology*. Oakland: University of California Press.

World Bank. 2018. *Country Partnership Framework for Burkina Faso for the Period FY18–FY23*. Washington DC: World Bank

Wouterse, Fleur. 2010. "Remittances, Poverty, Inequality and Welfare: Evidence from the Central Plateau of Burkina Faso." *The Journal of Development Studies* 46(4): 771–89.

Zeilig, Leo. 2017. "Burkina Faso: From Thomas Sankara to Popular Resistance." *Review of African Political Economy* 44(151): 155–64.

Zigon, Jarrett. 2018. "Hope and Waiting in Post-Soviet Moscow." In *Ethnographies of Waiting, Doubt, Hope and Uncertainty*, ed. Manpreet K. Janeja and Andreas Bandak, 65–86. London: Bloomsbury Academic.

Index

www.ingramcontent.com/pod-product-compliance
Ingram Content Group UK Ltd.
Pitfield, Milton Keynes, MK11 3LW, UK
UKHW021837150926
8656IPUK00004B/24

9 781805 391975